WHAT YOU MUST KNOW ABOUT

MEMORY LOSS

& HOW YOU CAN STOP IT

A GUIDE TO PROVEN TECHNIQUES AND SUPPLEMENTS TO MAINTAIN, STRENGTHEN, OR REGAIN MEMORY

Other Books
by Dr. Pamela Wartian Smith

What You Must Know About
Vitamins, Minerals, Herbs & More

What You Must Know About
Women's Hormones

Why You Can't Lose Weight

WHAT YOU MUST KNOW ABOUT

MEMORY LOSS

& HOW YOU CAN STOP IT

A GUIDE TO PROVEN TECHNIQUES AND SUPPLEMENTS TO MAINTAIN, STRENGTHEN, OR REGAIN MEMORY

PAMELA WARTIAN SMITH, MD, MPH

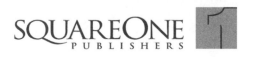

SQUAREONE
PUBLISHERS

EDITOR: R. M. Bromberg
COVER DESIGNER: Jeannie Tudor
TYPESETTER: Gary A. Rosenberg

The information and advice contained in this book are based upon the research and the personal and professional experiences of the author. They are not intended as a substitute for consulting with a healthcare professional. The publisher and author are not responsible for any adverse effects or consequences resulting from the use of any of the suggestions, preparations, or procedures discussed in this book. All matters pertaining to your physical health should be supervised by a healthcare professional. It is a sign of wisdom, not cowardice, to seek a second or third opinion.

Square One Publishers
115 Herricks Road
Garden City Park, NY 11040
(516) 535-2010 • (877) 900-BOOK
www.squareonepublishers.com

Library of Congress Cataloging-in-Publication Data

Smith, Pamela Wartian.
  What you must know about memory loss & how you can stop it / Pamela Wartian Smith, MD, MPH.
     pages cm
  Includes bibliographical references and index.
  ISBN 978-0-7570-0386-8
  1. Memory disorders. 2. Memory disorders—Patients—Rehabilitation. 3. Brain—Diseases—Treatment. I. Title.
  RC394.M46S65 2014
  616.8'3—dc23
                          2013043596

Printed in the United States of America

10   9   8   7   6   5   4   3   2   1

Contents

To Dr. Patricia Pierce,
whose contributions as a mother,
physician, and educator have been invaluable.
Her kindness, patience, and brilliance
will be missed.

Acknowledgments

To my publisher, Rudy Shur, whose hard work and dedication to this project were neverending.

To my editor, Miye Bromberg, who was willing to spend countless hours and days on this book, as the best editors do.

WHAT YOU MUST KNOW ABOUT
MEMORY LOSS & HOW YOU CAN STOP IT

Introduction

A t one point or another, most of us have experienced some form of memory loss. You forget where you left your cell phone, you open the refrigerator but suddenly can't remember what it was you were going to take out, or you can't recall the name of that great restaurant you visited last week! These little lapses are normal—and as we get older, these moments seem to become more common for most of us. This can be very frustrating, as our cognitive abilities are critical to making us who we are.

The fact is, aging can and does have an impact on our ability to remember. Fortunately, science has shown that most types of memory loss and cognitive impairment can be successfully treated, reversed, and even prevented. In the last thirty years, medical researchers have greatly ramped up their studies in this area. Scientists have investigated the factors that drive all forms of memory loss—from normal age-related memory impairment to dementia—and they have also looked at older individuals who have aged without losing their mental acuity. As a result, we have at our disposal a new wealth of information on memory loss. How can we put this information to work? What can we do to keep our minds sharp and accurate throughout our lives?

What You Must Know About Memory Loss & How You Can Stop It has reviewed thousands of studies to provide you with the most prevalent causes of memory loss and to offer real solutions to this growing problem. While the science behind many of these studies is complex, I have done my best to summarize each idea in plain English. Where scientific jargon must be used, it is accompanied by a clear explanation. In dealing with dementia and other related memory-robbing diseases, I have pro-

1

vided the most current information available. If you or your doctor wishes to look into any specific issues in more detail, I encourage you to consult the References section in the back of the book; there, I have cited the most important studies used to support the material in each chapter. My hope is to show you that solutions to memory loss are within your grasp.

The book begins by presenting you with the fundamentals you will need in order to understand why memory loss happens. Chapter 1 outlines the basic parts of the brain, detailing their functions in forming and maintaining memory. It also provides a general overview of the different types of memory and the three major categories of cognitive impairment.

The book is then divided into two parts. The purpose of Part I is to familiarize you with some of the most common sources of memory loss. Each chapter in Part I discusses a different factor that can potentially contribute to cognitive decline: cardiovascular disease, heavy metal poisoning, hormonal imbalance, inflammation, and insomnia are among the worst offenders. Every chapter is preceded by a questionnaire that will help you recognize whether the condition discussed within might be affecting you. If it is, you will want to read further. You will learn about the symptoms, causes, and risk factors of that condition, and then you will find out how it is typically diagnosed and treated.

Part I also includes a chapter on dementia, the most severe form of memory loss. Currently, most forms of dementia are considered to be both unpreventable and nonreversible—that is, they cannot be avoided or cured. Still, there are many things you can do to treat the symptoms and even minimize your risk of developing Alzheimer's disease and other dementias. As research is ongoing, my intent is to give you the most up-to-date information available so that you will be aware of your options in managing these devastating and increasingly common diseases.

While Part I discusses specific problems that cause memory loss, Part II serves as a more general guide to memory maintenance and enhancement. Each of the first five chapters in Part II features a lifestyle factor that is critical to keeping your mind in peak condition: physical activity, mental activity, sleep, stress management, and diet. By getting more sleep and exercise, keeping your mind active, minimizing your stress, and eating a wholesome diet, you will be better able to stave off any cognitive decline. You may even feel quicker and more alert! In addition, you might want to try adding a nutritional supplement to your daily routine. The last chapter provides a summary of the nutritional supplements shown to be most effective in improving your recall and focus. Although there is no "miracle drug" that will magically make you the intellectual equivalent of Albert Einstein, the supplements discussed in Chapter 13 have been shown to produce modest but significant benefits for those who consume them.

It really is possible to keep your mind sharp and focused throughout your lifespan, but it will not happen without a commitment on your part. In picking up this book, you have taken the important first step toward optimizing your cognition and memory. Now it's time to take the next steps. To find out how to make the most of your brain and take care of it for years to come, continue reading!

1

The Brain and Memory Loss

A man's real possession is his memory.
In nothing else is he rich, in nothing else is he poor.
—Alexander Smith, nineteenth-century Scottish poet

Most of us are instinctively familiar with the idea of memory loss. All of us have forgotten an important piece of information at one time or another. But what is actually happening in your brain when you find yourself searching for answers? And how do you distinguish normal, temporary memory impairment from more serious and permanent cognitive decline?

This chapter provides a basic overview of memory and memory loss. First, you will be introduced to your brain, learning about its parts and their functions in forming and maintaining memory. Building on this foundation of knowledge, the chapter then details the different types of memory. Finally, you will learn about the three major categories of memory loss. By learning how to distinguish between these different conditions, you will be better able to recognize and treat cognitive decline in yourself or a loved one.

THE BRAIN

Your brain is the most important organ in your body. Although it accounts for only 2 percent of your body weight, the brain uses 25 to 50 percent of all the calories and oxygen you take in. Modulating your thoughts, emotions, actions, sensations, and memories, your brain is the one thing that makes you who you are.

Because it is responsible for so many different functions, your brain is by far the most complex organ in your body. It is composed of over 100 billion *neurons* (nerve cells) and a trillion *glial cells*, sometimes called support cells because they amplify and sustain the actions of the neurons. Neurons communicate with each other by transmitting electrical signals through special points of contact called *synapses*. Chemicals called *neurotransmitters* help conduct these signals through the synapses, allowing them to move at lightning speeds around your brain. When you learn or form memories, your neurons are building new pathways for the electrical signals to travel—literally creating new associations between your brain cells!

It is this connectivity that makes it possible for us to accumulate and retain a vast and varied quantity of information. Each of your neurons can potentially link to thousands of other neurons; by some estimates, almost a million connections are formed every second! Over time, however, these connections can weaken or disappear, resulting in lost memories or information. When you sleep, your brain also "prunes" these connections, weakening or destroying connections that are no longer essential; this allows your mind to conserve energy and keep a narrower focus on the memories that are still useful. Pathways can also shift or get "rerouted," altering existing memories or information. The important thing to understand is that your brain is constantly changing; new connections and even new neurons can be generated well into old age. This capacity for change—a phenomenon scientists call *neuroplasticity*—is good news, since it suggests that there are many things you can do to help keep your memory and focus sharp.

The brain is composed of three main structural components: the brain stem, the cerebellum, and the cerebrum.

- The *brain stem* connects the brain to the spinal cord, and thus to the rest of your body. It controls your reflexes and many of your vital and involuntary (automatic or unconscious) body functions, including breathing, digestion, and blood circulation.

- The *cerebellum*, nicknamed the "little brain," is a small, wrinkled knob of tissue found towards the back of the head, under the cerebrum. It primarily serves to integrate sensory information from your eyes, ears, and muscles in order to coordinate movement and maintain balance.

- The *cerebrum* is the part most of us envision when we think about the brain. Weighing about three pounds, it is the soft, jelly-like mass that takes up most of the space in your skull. More extensively developed in humans than in any other mammal, the cerebrum is responsible for much of our higher functioning, including emotion, thoughts, personality, and memory. It also controls voluntary (conscious) movement.

  Your cerebrum is divided straight down the middle into two halves, or *hemispheres*—right and left. Generally speaking, the left hemisphere controls the right side of your body, and the right hemisphere controls the left. Both hemispheres are further subdivided into special lobes, each of which has a specific function.

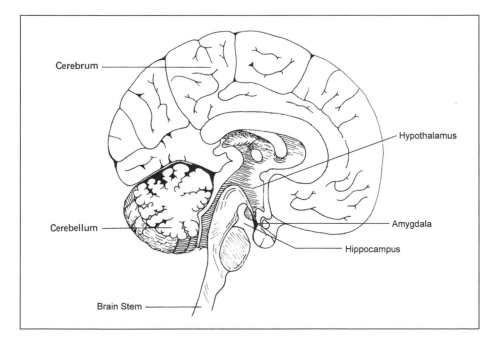

Figure 1.1. **Parts of the brain**
Human brain as seen when cut into equal right and left halves.

- The *frontal lobes* control your ability to think, plan, reason, and imagine, and are integral to short-term memory construction and motor movement. On the left frontal lobe is a region called the *Broca's area*, which is responsible for transforming thoughts into words. The *parietal lobes* process certain forms of sensory input—touch, taste, temperature —and, with the cerebellum, help coordinate movement and perception of spatial relationships. They also seem to play a role in establishing an understanding of symbolic or mathematical information. The *occipital lobes* are primarily associated with processing visual input; among other functions, they connect new visual stimuli to other images stored in your memory. Finally, the *temporal lobes* interpret smells, sounds, and certain tastes. They are also the lobes that are most heavily associated with the processing of emotions and memory.

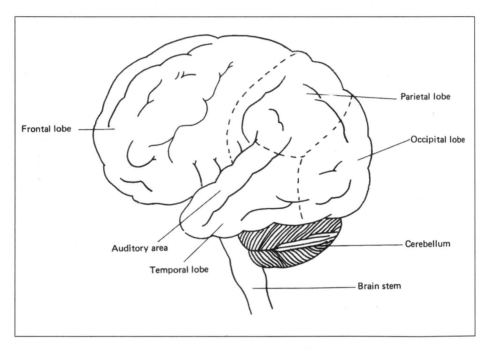

Figure 1.2. **Lobes of the brain**
Surface view of the right side of the brain. The lobes of the cerebral hemisphere
are separated by dashed lines.

In addition to the three main parts of your brain, there is another small component that has enormous impact on your focus and recall—the limbic system. Located under your cerebrum, deep in your inner brain, the limbic system is a collection of brain structures that are primarily responsible for learning, emotions, and memory. As with the lobes of the cerebrum, these structures occur in symmetrical pairs, one in each hemisphere. Of these structures, the most important are the hypothalamus, the amygdala, and the hippocampus.

- The *hypothalamus* serves as an intermediary between your nervous system and your endocrine (hormone-producing) system. It produces hormones that regulate many vital functions, including hunger and satiety, sleep and consciousness, sex drive, body temperature, and mood. The *amygdala* processes emotions, particularly fear, anxiety, and anger; it also plays a role in modulating (altering) long-term memories in response to these emotions.

- Perhaps most important for our interests, the limbic system also houses the *hippocampus,* your brain's memory center. The hippocampus is a small, crescent-shaped tube that is responsible for both the formation of new memories and the conversion of short-term (momentary) memories into long-term (lasting) memories. The hippocampus is particularly vulnerable to injury; when it is damaged by stress or Alzheimer's disease, people start to lose their ability to create or retain memories. Because of the central role played by the hippocampus in memory, scientists are constantly trying to pinpoint the exact mechanisms that guide its actions; a better understanding of the hippocampus could prove the key to curing memory loss.

Now that you have a better sense of the major components of the brain and their roles in memory and cognition, let's take a closer look at the different types of memory.

TYPES OF MEMORY

As you probably realize, there are many different kinds of memories, allowing you to draw upon many different kinds of experiences and learned information. The broadest way to categorize memories is by duration, or how long the memory lasts.

Sensory Memory

Sensory memories are the briefest of all memories. Lasting less than a second, sensory memories are instantaneous perceptions of things you are currently seeing, hearing, smelling, tasting, or touching. Sensory memories are processed automatically—almost unconsciously—as you go about daily life. Sensory memories that your brain evaluates as important or significant get passed into your short-term memory for further consideration.

Short-term and Working Memory

Primarily associated with your frontal and parietal lobes, your *short-term memory* (STM) holds a small number of memories for a slightly longer period, lasting anywhere from a few seconds up to a minute. Short-term memory is a form of *working memory*, so called because it retains information that you access immediately in order to operate fluidly on a moment-to-moment basis.

Working memory creates associations between events that occurred in the very recent past, allowing you to plan and execute various tasks. For example, working memory makes it possible for you to speak in full sentences: by remembering how you began a sentence ("I saw Mark today"), you're able to finish it (". . .and he said you were coming to the meeting tonight."). Or it can allow you to remember directions that you've just been given ("To get to the museum, take a right at the next block, walk three blocks, then take a left at 53rd Street and walk two more.")

Your working memory holds memories that are temporary and largely functional in nature. Short-term memory has a fairly limited capacity; typically, you can retain about seven different pieces of information—for example, the digits in a phone number—for about ten to fifteen seconds. By repeating this information over and over to yourself (a process called *rehearsal*), you can increase the number of seconds you're able to remember a piece of information—giving you just enough time to type that number into your phone.

Ordinarily, as soon as you've used a memory to perform a task, the memory decays, or fades from your mind, because it is no longer needed. (In neurological terms, the electrical signal stops flowing between neurons, and the new pathway on which it traveled gradually disappears.) As a result, a spot opens up in your short-term memory, allowing a new piece of information to take its place. If all the slots in your short-term memory are occupied, these different memories can compete for your attention, producing the impression that you are "juggling" different thoughts at the same time, and making it a challenge to focus on any one of them specifically. When your attention is thus divided, you will also have more difficulty *encoding* all these memories in the first place—that is, taking in information and turning it into either short-term or long-term memories. This is why it's hard for you to recall where you just put your car keys if you took them out of your bag while simultaneously texting one friend to meet you at the movies and trying to remember the address of the theater.

Sometimes your short-term memories don't immediately disappear after use. If a short-term memory is deemed to be important, it can be stabilized and converted into a long-term memory.

Long-term Memory

Capable of holding vast amounts of information for unlimited periods of time, your *long-term memory* (LTM) is potentially the most powerful of all your memory stores. Scientists are not sure of the exact mechanisms by which memories are *consolidated,* or transferred from short-term to long-term memory. As discussed earlier, many believe that the process involves strengthening, reinforcing, or rerouting neural pathways or networks that are established during the initial phase of short-term memory construction. It's also possible that consolidation entails the creation of entirely new pathways, or the elimination of old and inefficient ones. The hippocampus plays an essential role in consolidation, acting as a sort of editor, sorting through most types of short-term memories and deciding which information will be stored in your long-term memory and which will be discarded.

While many long-term memories may seem to be "permanently" fixed in your mind, in fact, recent research indicates that many of these memories can change over time, in response to new input or re-evaluation. Unlike short-term memory, which primarily involves the frontal and parietal lobes, long-term memory can potentially engage and connect any area of the brain   and thus be altered or adapted as well.

There are several different forms of long-term memory.

Declarative Memories

Declarative memories are what we usually think of when we think about memories—they're memories that you recall consciously or explicitly. There are two main types of declarative memories, both of which engage the hippocampus and parts of the temporal lobe. *Episodic memories* are mental records of episodes, or events, in your life: that time six years ago when you went to Rome with your husband for your anniversary, or the conversation you had with Peter Manning at the carwash on Sunday. *Semantic memories* tend to deal with facts and other word-based information: for example, that Kampala is the capital of Uganda, or that an ostrich is a type of flightless bird. Semantic memories are often reinforced or informed by episodic memories: for example, by remembering exactly where in your house you sat when you read this chapter, you may be better able to recall the types of memory described within.

Nondeclarative Memories

Nondeclarative memories are memories that you recall unconsciously or implicitly. They are sometimes called *procedural memories,* because these memories are formed by repeat experience and enable automatic actions or behaviors: driving a car, for example, or throwing a football. Once you've learned how to change a light bulb, it becomes a nearly permanent nondeclarative memory; you never have to consciously consider how you go about the process. Nondeclarative memories seem to bypass the hippocampus and temporal lobes, instead involving more local neural networks in the cerebellum and the frontal lobes. This is why people who have damage to the hippocampus—like many patients with Alzheimer's disease—are often perfectly capable of performing certain routine tasks that they had learned to do previously, such as peeling an apple or brushing their teeth.

Having learned about both the structures of the brain and the various types of memory, we now have a good foundation for understanding the different forms of memory loss.

TYPES OF MEMORY LOSS

While most of us think of dementia when we are asked to identify typical memory loss, there are actually three main categories or levels of memory loss, which differ in severity and responsiveness to treatment.

Age-Related Memory Impairment (AMI)

Age-related memory impairment describes the mild forgetfulness that occurs as a natural consequence of the aging process. According to some estimates, the capacity and acuity of human memory peaks at the age of twenty-five; by the time you are seventy-five, your memory has declined by an average total of 43 percent. This is because as you grow older, certain physical and chemical changes take place in your brain as a matter of course. By some estimates, your brain can shrink by as much as 15 percent as a normal part of the aging process; the hippocampus alone can atrophy at a rate of 1 to 2 percent each year in older adults. Additionally, your neurons themselves will start to shrink and lose function, connections between neurons weaken, and production of the neurotransmitters that transmit electrical signals decreases.

AMI is by far the most minor form of memory loss, and also the most common, affecting about 40 percent of all people aged 65 or older, or about 16 million people. It is considered to be a benign condition; that is, its effects are temporary and don't affect your general ability to live your daily life. Episodic memory is the form of memory most significantly affected by normal aging; this is why, for example, older people have a harder time remembering what they ate for dinner two nights earlier.

AMI can also incur temporary lapses in short-term memory recall, resulting in what many people call "brain farts" or "senior moments": for a second, you forget where you put your handbag, or when your boss appears you can't remember what it was you meant to tell her, or all of a sudden you can't bring to mind the name of the person you want to talk about. You snap your fingers, rack your brain, or say, "It's on the tip of my tongue!" Generally, the information will come back to you fairly quickly.

Not all of the mental changes associated with aging are bad. Studies have shown that certain areas of cognition actually improve with age, including semantic memory, or the ability to recall general facts and concepts. And most of the time, any cognitive decline that occurs as a result of age tends not to be serious; some people will never see any appreciable decline in their mental abilities at all, their minds staying razor-sharp well into their eighties or nineties.

Moreover, age-related memory impairment is easy to treat—and even reverse—due to its transient and relatively negligible nature. Often, it can be effectively reduced or even eliminated simply by addressing the factors that increase the rate at which your brain ages—including stress, insomnia, poor psychological health, lack of physical exercise, hormonal decline and imbalances, inflammation, exposure to toxins, and poor nutrition. This book seeks to show you how to identify and manage these factors, so that you will always enjoy good mental focus and recall.

Mild Cognitive Impairment (MCI)

Only recently identified by researchers, mild cognitive impairment (MCI) is considered to be an intermediate stage between normal age-related memory impairment and full-fledged dementia. It involves a decline in memory and cognitive function that is somewhat more noticeable than that of AMI—though, as with AMI, this decline is never so severe that it disrupts daily life. Incidents of forgetting take place more frequently, and it takes longer to recall certain words, facts, or events. Although it is sometimes difficult to distinguish MCI from AMI, patients with MCI often have problems with balance and coordination that do not occur in subjects with normal age-related memory loss.

MCI is also characterized by a higher degree of damage to the brain and neurons. Autopsies of patients with MCI reveal moderate atrophy or shrinkage of the hippocampus and temporal lobes, and more widespread amyloid plaques and neurofibrillary tangles, two types of brain growths that can obstruct or inhibit brain activity and are associated with the development of Alzheimer's disease.

Because these types of brain damage are identical to—though less extensive than—those that characterize the various forms of dementia, MCI is often considered to be an early or transitional stage of dementia itself. According to one study, of the 10 percent of people aged sixty-five or older who have MCI, nearly 15 percent go on to develop Alzheimer's disease each year. At the very least, MCI constitutes a major risk factor for Alzheimer's disease and other forms of dementia; that is, having MCI significantly increases your risk of developing these more serious conditions. Nonetheless, many people with MCI never progress to dementia, and some recover or even improve cognitive function once properly diagnosed and treated.

Unfortunately, there are no tools that can predict the specific outcome of this condition in an individual. There are also no formal criteria for diagnosing MCI. Typically, you or your family will be conscious of an increasing difficulty remembering, planning, multitasking, following instructions, or making decisions. You may find yourself repeating yourself more frequently, or getting lost even when you know the area well. If MCI is suspected, your doctor may assess your mental status by having you take tests to evaluate your memory and judgment. Your doctor may also perform certain neurological checks in order to determine how well your brain and nervous system are working, evaluating your sensory processing, reflexes, balance, and coordination.

Risk factors for MCI are nearly identical to those for age-related memory impairment, but also include diabetes, smoking, and high blood pressure. Patients who have MCI are also more likely to have a genetic variation called apolipoprotein E-e4 (APOE-e4), although having this variation does not mean that you will necessarily suffer MCI or Alzheimer's disease, with which it is also associated.

Currently, there are no medications to treat mild cognitive impairment. The good news is that, as with age-related memory impairment, by managing the risk factors that exacerbate or contribute to MCI, you can effectively minimize or even reverse this form of memory loss and cognitive decline. This book will show you how.

Dementia

Dementia is a general term for cognitive decline so severe that it interferes with daily life. It involves wide-ranging and often progressive loss of brain function, as many of the neurological changes initiated in mild cognitive impairment become more pronounced or extensive. Symptoms can include significant memory loss, lack of focus, impaired judgment and reasoning, difficulty planning and organizing, mood swings, paranoia, disorientation, delusions, inappropriate behavior, personality shifts, and an inability to communicate or understand language.

Dementia is common, particularly among people over sixty-five years of age. A recent study estimates that almost 6.8 million Americans have dementia, with about 1.8 million of those severely affected. While age itself does not *cause* dementia, it is the condition's single greatest risk factor. That is, the older you are, the more likely it is that you will develop some form of dementia—studies find that almost half of all Americans age eighty-five or older are afflicted. It's important to understand, however, that dementia is not a natural part of the aging process, plenty of people live long lives without ever developing any cognitive issues.

There are many different forms of dementia, each distinguished by a particular type of brain damage. For more information on these specific conditions, see Chapters 2 and 7.

Alzheimer's Disease

Alzheimer's disease (AD) is the most common type of dementia, affecting at least 5.2 million Americans and accounting for an estimated 60 to 80 percent of all dementia cases. It is characterized by a sharp decline in the production of key neurotransmitter acetylcholine, and by the unchecked cerebral growth of two forms of protein deposits—beta-amyloid plaques and neurofibrillary (tau) tangles. Scientists are unsure whether these factors cause Alzheimer's disease, or are themselves the results of an underlying problem, but their presence is associated with the widespread death or dysfunction of neurons, resulting in brain atrophy and shrinkage.

Alzheimer's is a progressive disease, meaning that damage to the cerebrum and hippocampus gradually worsens over time; protein deposits can begin to grow as early as twenty years before any symptoms are seen. AD involves a severe deterioration of thinking skills and memory. Episodic memory is the first to be affected, followed by short-term, semantic, and procedural memory. As the disease advances, nearly all brain functions are affected; eventually, even physical processes like swallowing or bowel control can become impaired. Though Alzheimer's disease is the subject of intense research, there is currently no known cure.

Vascular Dementia (VaD)

Vascular dementia (VaD), sometimes called multi-infarct dementia, is the second most common type of dementia in the United States, accounting for 20 to 30 percent of all dementia cases. It is defined as a decline in thinking skills and memory caused by interrupted blood flow to the brain, often as the result of a stroke or series of strokes. Because its symptoms often appear progressively and can mimic or even coexist with those of Alzheimer's disease, vascular dementia sometimes goes undiagnosed or misdiagnosed. Symptoms of vascular dementia vary according to the area of the brain affected by the loss of blood flow, but tend to manifest initially in the form of confusion and impaired judgment; memory loss is common but not necessarily present. Vascular dementia differs from the other major forms of dementia in that it is partially preventable; by controlling the risk factors that contribute to heart disease, you can significantly reduce the likelihood that you will ever suffer from this disease. For more information, see Chapter 2.

Dementia with Lewy Bodies (DLB)

Dementia with Lewy bodies (DLB) is the third most common type of dementia, accounting for 10 to 25 percent of all cases. It is characterized by the cerebral presence of Lewy bodies, certain protein clumps that are found in other neurodegenerative disorders, most notably Parkinson's disease and, to a lesser degree, Alzheimer's disease. Because of this shared factor, DLB bears some resemblance to both diseases, entailing

Alzheimer-like cognitive decline, but also Parkinsonian motor issues such as muscle rigidity and body tremors. Dementia with Lewy bodies can also be distinguished from other forms of dementia in that its most prominent symptoms include visual hallucinations, fluctuations in alertness and focus, and sleep disorders; memory loss may or may not occur. Currently, there is no cure for DLB.

Frontotemporal Dementia (FTD)

Frontotemporal dementia (FTD) describes a relatively rare group of disorders that primarily affect the frontal and temporal lobes. While it accounts for between 10 to 15 percent of all dementia cases, it is disproportionately common among younger patients, accounting for 20 to 50 percent of all dementia cases in people aged sixty-five or less. Its early onset—patients are usually diagnosed around age fifty-seven, thirteen years before the average Alzheimer's patient—is usually the best clue in identifying this disease. FTD is also more likely to involve changes in behavior and speech than Alzheimer's disease, with memory loss less common at the outset. Frontotemporal dementia is believed to stem mainly from inherited genetic mutations, although in addition it is often characterized by the presence of microscopic protein structures called Pick bodies. Currently, there is no cure for frontotemporal dementia.

Mixed Dementia

Mixed dementia is a medical state in which different forms of dementia occur at the same time. It most frequently refers to the coexistence of Alzheimer's disease and vascular dementia, but can also describe cases in which dementia with Lewy bodies coexists with Alzheimer's disease. Mixed dementia also acknowledges the fact that some forms of dementia are characterized by (and might stem from) the same brain abnormalities; for example, Lewy bodies can be found in both Alzheimer's and DLB patients. A recently identified disease, mixed dementia is rarely diagnosed during a patient's life; only an autopsy can confirm the simultaneous presence of the brain abnormalities that characterize the different forms of dementia.

Other Types of Dementia

In addition to the major types of dementia discussed above, dementia can be caused by various other diseases or conditions, including Parkinson's disease, Huntington's disease, Creutzfeldt-Jakob disease, HIV/

AIDS, Wernicke-Korsakoff syndrome, alcohol abuse, and traumatic brain injury. In these cases, dementia is essentially a symptom of a larger problem; accordingly, treatment for these forms usually depends on the underlying disease or condition.

Because dementia is a complex phenomenon whose causes and risk factors are still not well understood, treatment options are limited. What makes dementia so insidious is the fact that it is almost always unpreventable and nonreversible: it can be managed, and even slowed by medication, but not cured. There are some exceptions to this rule, as when dementia is caused by external and removable factors, such as infections, nutritional deficiencies, dehydration, metabolic and endocrine dysfunction, immune disorders, reactions to medications, exposure to certain heavy metals, oxygen deprivation, thyroid disorders, or brain tumors.

Still, while new theories and treatments are being developed, there is much you can do to offset or reduce the controllable risk factors associated with the onset or progression of dementia. This book focuses on many of those factors, showing you how to improve your diet, sleep, stress levels, and physical and mental activity, so that you may help protect yourself from serious memory loss. For a specific look at dementia and what you can do about it, see Chapter 7.

CONCLUSION

Memory loss is a daunting prospect to many people, but it shouldn't be. Knowledge is power. In reading this chapter, you have taken a critical first step toward optimizing your mental acuity and focus. Now that you understand how the brain works and what the various types of memory and memory loss are, you will be better equipped to identify—and treat—any cognitive decline that you or a loved one might experience. Moreover, you will find this foundation of knowledge useful as you continue to peruse the rest of the book, particularly as specific causes of memory loss are presented.

PART I

THE PROBLEMS

Is Your Memory Loss Caused by Cardiovascular Disease?

QUESTIONNAIRE

This test was designed to help you determine whether cardiovascular disease might be affecting your memory and cognition. Read each question carefully and place a check mark in the box that best represents your answer.

	Yes	No	Unsure
1. Do you eat foods that are high in sodium (salt)?	☐	☐	☐
2. Do you eat foods that are high in saturated fats?	☐	☐	☐
3. Are you overweight by twenty pounds or more?	☐	☐	☐
4. Do you lead a sedentary life?	☐	☐	☐
5. Do you smoke?	☐	☐	☐
6. Do you drink more than one serving of alcohol a day?	☐	☐	☐
7. Do you experience chest pains on a regular basis?	☐	☐	☐
8. Do you suffer from chronic shortness of breath?	☐	☐	☐
9. Do your arms, hands or legs often feel numb, weak, or cold?	☐	☐	☐
10. Do you often feel dizzy or experience fainting spells?	☐	☐	☐

If you answered "yes" to the majority of these questions, you may be at risk for heart disease—and the poor circulation that can cause memory loss!

2

Cardiovascular Disease

Few people realize that memory loss and heart disease are related—but they can be. Dementia and even forgetfulness may be directly caused by cardiovascular disease. How so? The connection is quite simple. Certain heart conditions reduce the normal flow of blood to the brain. In atherosclerosis, your blood vessels can get clogged due to the buildup of plaque. High blood pressure can damage or cause leaks in your blood vessels, and low blood pressure can also simply prevent sufficient blood from reaching your brain. When your brain's blood supply is thus cut off or limited, your brain no longer gets the oxygen and nutrients it needs to carry out all your essential cognitive processes.

Over time, this deficiency of oxygen and nutrients can cause forgetfulness and mild confusion. Should your brain cells be deprived of oxygen altogether for more than a few seconds—because of a heart attack or a stroke—they can die, causing permanent damage to your cerebral cortex. One of the results of this damage is a progressive impairment or loss of brain function—a condition called vascular dementia.

Hopefully you will never suffer from vascular dementia, or from the heart attack or stroke that often precede it! But by understanding that memory loss can be a symptom of an underlying cardiovascular condition, you may be able to remedy the problem before it progresses. The questionnaire at the beginning of this chapter is designed to help you determine whether heart disease might be the source of memory loss for you or your loved ones. If you answered "yes" to many of the questions, then you may be at risk for cardiovascular disease. Read on to learn how to recognize your heart condition, acknowledge its risk factors and causes, and take steps to treat and correct it. By improving your blood circulation, you may very well be able to reduce or prevent against memory loss and cognitive decline.

So that you may be able to identify any heart problem before it worsens, let's first look at the symptoms most commonly associated with poor circulation and cardiovascular disease.

SYMPTOMS OF CARDIOVASCULAR DISEASE

There are many forms of cardiovascular disease, all of which can potentially affect the flow of blood to the brain. Although symptoms for specific heart conditions can vary, there are three more general markers that indicate that your blood circulation is not as strong as it should be:

- Chest pain (angina)

- Shortness of breath

- Hands and feet that are painful or feel cold, numb, or weak

You may also experience any of the following symptoms:

- Dizziness

- Fainting spells

- Fatigue

- Indigestion

- Nausea

- Pain or discomfort in the upper abdomen

- Pain or discomfort in the shoulder or back

- Pain or discomfort in the jaw or neck

If you have suffered from any of these symptoms, you may be at risk for cardiovascular disease, and should consult your healthcare provider. But be forewarned; many people who have cardiovascular disease experience no obvious symptoms. More often than not, women do not experience severe symptoms like chest pain; instead, they may suffer more nonspecific symptoms such as fatigue or nausea, making early diagnosis difficult.

CAUSES OF CARDIOVASCULAR DISEASE

Why do some people develop poor blood circulation? While there are many forms of heart disease, there are three primary cardiovascular conditions that cause your blood flow to be reduced or limited. The first is atherosclerosis, a condition in which your arteries are narrowed or clogged by plaque, restricting the amount of blood that can travel through your system. The second is high blood pressure (hypertension), in which your heart propels blood with such force that your arteries and veins can tear, creating holes in your blood vessels through which the blood will leak out instead of traveling on to your brain. And finally, circulation can be reduced by low blood pressure (hypotension), a condition in which your heart doesn't pump blood through your system with enough force, producing a weak and inadequate flow of blood to your brain and other organs.

What causes these three critical cardiovascular conditions?

Causes of Atherosclerosis

- Diabetes
- High cholesterol
- High blood pressure (hypertension)
- Smoking

Causes of High Blood Pressure (Hypertension)

- Congenital (birth) defects in blood vessels
- Drugs (including alcohol, birth control pills, certain cold medications, decongestants, diuretics, certain migraine medications, and painkillers)
- Endocrine conditions (acromegaly, Cushing's syndrome, overactive or underactive thyroid)
- Heredity
- Illegal drugs (cocaine, amphetamines)
- Kidney conditions
- Obesity
- Pregnancy

Causes of Low Blood Pressure (Hypotension)

- Anaphylaxis (severe allergic reaction)
- Anemia
- Dehydration
- Diabetes
- Drugs (including alcohol, alpha and beta blockers, diuretics, certain anti-anxiety medications and antidepressants, heart medicines, and painkillers)

- Endocrine conditions (under-active or overactive thyroid)

- Pre-existing heart conditions (heart attack, heart failure, heart valve problems, low heart rate)

- Pregnancy

- Reduced blood volume (as result of dehydration, starvation, or hemorrhage)

Although it is not always possible to pinpoint the specific cause of each case of atherosclerosis or abnormal blood pressure, the conditions and drugs listed above represent some of the most common sources of these heart ailments. Next, we'll explore the factors that put you at greater risk for developing heart disease.

RISK FACTORS FOR CARDIOVASCULAR DISEASE

Many different factors contribute to your risk for cardiovascular disease. Some, like your family history, are beyond your control. Others, like diet, are the result of poor or unhealthy lifestyle choices. Below is a list of risk factors that may raise the likelihood that you will develop heart disease.

Uncontrollable Factors

- **Age**. Your risk increases as you get older.

- **Sex**. Men generally have a greater risk for heart disease. Women's risk increases after menopause to equal or surpass that of similarly-aged men.

- **Heredity**. Race and family history of heart disease can affect risk; African Americans, Mexican Americans, American Indians, native Hawaiians, and some Asian Americans have higher risks of heart disease than do Caucasians.

Controllable Factors

- High blood pressure

- High blood cholesterol (especially high LDL cholesterol)

- High homocysteine levels

- Gum disease

- Diabetes

- Obesity

- Physical inactivity

- Poor diet (high sodium intake)

- Smoking

- Stress

If you suffer from any of the risk factors listed above, you may have a higher risk for heart disease and poor circulation, and should consult with a healthcare provider for counsel and treatment options. The following section will show you the methods by which doctors most often diagnose heart disease.

TESTS USED TO DIAGNOSE CARDIOVASCULAR DISEASE

Doctors use many tests to determine whether you have (or are at risk for) cardiovascular disease. While the specific type of test used will depend on the condition you are suspected of having, the following is a general list of the diagnostic tools most frequently used to diagnose the most common heart conditions associated with poor circulation.

Tests Used to Diagnose Atherosclerosis

- **Artery imaging tests**. A variety of imaging tools can be used with or without dye injection to provide a more detailed look at your arteries, revealing aneurysms, calcium deposits, and any hardened or narrowed areas. Tools include cardiac catheterization and angiogram, computerized tomography (CT) scans, and magnetic resonance angiography (MRA).

- **Blood test**. Measures cholesterol and blood sugar levels.

- **Electrocardiogram (ECG)**. Measures your heart's electrical activity. Can be used with stress test.

- **Physical examination**. Can expose evidence for narrowed or hardened arteries, including weak pulse, decreased blood pressure, abnormal blood flow, or aneurysm.

- **Stress (exercise) test**. Measures your heart's performance under physical duress (a jog or bike ride).

Tests Used to Diagnose High or Low Blood Pressure (Hypertension and Hypotension)

- **Blood pressure test**. Using a stethoscope and an inflatable rubber cuff, readings are taken of both systolic blood pressure (pressure on artery walls when heart contracts) and diastolic blood pressure (pressure on artery walls when heart relaxes).

- **Blood test**. Measures cholesterol levels.

- **Electrocardiogram (ECG)**. Measures heart's electrical activity.

LIFESTYLE CHANGES

Although there are many risk factors for cardiovascular disease that are beyond your control, there are many others that can be controlled by making good choices for your general health. Thus any initiative to improve or prevent heart disease should begin with an evaluation of your lifestyle, as presented with the questionnaire at the beginning of the chapter. Do you eat a lot of foods that are high in fats and salt? Are you overweight or obese? Do you lead a sedentary life? Do you smoke? Do you drink to excess? If you answered "yes" to any of those questions, your lifestyle puts you at risk for heart disease.

Fortunately, it is relatively simple to make changes to your habits in order to minimize your cardiovascular risk. This section outlines the most important ways that you can reduce your likelihood of developing heart disease without (or in addition to) medication or surgical intervention: adopt a well-balanced diet, maintain a healthy weight, exercise, manage stress levels, stop smoking, and avoid or limit alcohol consumption. By following these simple guidelines, you can improve your blood circulation, and help mitigate or even prevent memory loss.

- **Avoid or Limit Alcohol Consumption**. Research indicates that moderate consumption—one beer, 4 ounces of wine, or 1.5 ounces of 80- or 100-proof spirits each day for women, or twice those volumes for men—may lower your risk of developing heart disease. But alcohol drunk in excess of these amounts can significantly raise your risk, increasing your triglyceride levels and contributing to high blood pressure, arrhythmia, and heart failure. So be careful not to overdo it!

- **Exercise**. Regular exercise is one of the best ways to reduce your risk of heart disease. It can help lower your cholesterol and blood pressure, and is a vital component of any plan to lose or maintain a healthy weight. Moreover, physical activity improves your body's ability to take in and use oxygen, and can strengthen and dilate your blood vessels—two benefits that have direct consequences for preventing against vascular dementia. For more information, see Chapter 8.

- **Maintain a Healthy Weight**. People who are overweight (having a body mass index, or BMI, of 25.0 to 29.9) or obese (having a BMI over 30.0) are at greater risk for developing heart disease. Accordingly, you should always try to maintain a healthy weight through exercise, proper diet, and other measures. If you have changed your lifestyle and still have trouble lowering or maintaining your weight, see a metabolic medicine specialist to determine the cause of your inability to lose weight. Your hormones may be out of balance, you may have allergies, or you might suffer a neurotransmitter dysfunction that prevents you from losing weight and keeping it off. If you are already overweight or obese, try to get back within a normal weight range. As the CDC reports, a loss of just 5 to 10 percent of your body weight can significantly decrease your likelihood of developing heart disease.

- **Manage Stress Levels**. Prolonged or high levels of stress can contribute to your risk of cardiovascular disease by raising your blood pressure and heart rate, causing irregular heart rhythms, damaging your arteries, and weakening your immune system. Accordingly, take steps to minimize the number and force of stressors in your life. For more information on how to manage stress, see Chapter 11.

- **Stop Smoking**. According to the American Heart Association, smoking is the most preventable cause of premature death in the United States, as it is associated with higher risk for many cardiovascular disorders, including atherosclerosis, heart attack, and stroke. Smoking— or even breathing in secondhand smoke—depletes your body's stores of good (HDL) cholesterol, temporarily raises your blood pressure, damages the lining of your blood vessels, decreases your circulation, and encourages the formation of dangerous blood clots. It also inhibits your ability to exercise, as the damage it does to your lungs makes it harder for you to breathe properly while you are exerting yourself. As the Cleveland Clinic has stated, there is no safe level of smoking; your risk for heart disease increases the longer you smoke and the more cigarettes you use each day. If you smoke; quit; if you do not smoke, limit your exposure to people who do.

ADOPT A WELL-BALANCED DIET

A wholesome, well-balanced diet is one of the cornerstones of good cardiovascular health. A good diet will not only lower your risk of heart disease more generally, but can also help you control other factors that contribute to its development, reducing cholesterol levels and decreasing your risk for obesity, high blood pressure, and diabetes.

While there are many specific diets that can improve your heart health, many doctors and scientists currently advocate the Mediterranean diet. A 2013 study conducted by the Harvard School of Public Health showed that this diet reduced risk of heart attack, stroke, and death from heart disease, by as much as 30 percent—a figure that is roughly equivalent to the use of a single statin drug. You will find a full overview of the Mediterranean diet in Chapter 12.

By following the guidelines provided, you may be able to reduce the likelihood that you will develop heart disease. If you already have a heart condition, eating a well-balanced diet like the one described in Chapter 12 can help prevent the recurrence of a heart attack or stroke. In addition, you should avoid eating foods to which you are allergic or have a sensitivity or intolerance; studies show that the allergic response can increase blood pressure. Eating a wholesome, well-balanced diet will allow your blood circulation to improve—and that's good news for your memory!

SUPPLEMENTS

For better cardiovascular health, you may also choose to incorporate one or more of the following supplements into your daily routine.

Supplement	Dosage	Considerations
Arginine	3,000 to 9,000 mg once a day.	Consult with your healthcare provider if you have kidney disease, liver disease, or herpes.
Berberine	300 to 500 mg three times a day.	
Carnitine	1,000 to 2,000 mg once a day.	Consult with your healthcare provider before taking if you have kidney or liver disease.
Coenzyme Q_{10}	120 to 400 mg once a day.	May reduce the effects of blood thinners. May cause diarrhea in dosages above 100 mg once a day.
D-ribose	5 to 30 g once a day.	May interact with insulin and diabetes medications.
Hawthorn	160 to 900 mg once a day.	May interfere with the absorption of some blood pressure medications. See your healthcare provider.

Supplement	Dosage	Considerations
Magnesium	600 to 800 mg once a day.	Not recommended for people with kidney disease. Reduce dosage if you experience diarrhea. Discontinue use and see healthcare provider if you experience abdominal pain.
Omega-3 fatty acids EPA/DHA (fish oil)	2,000 to 3,000 mg once a day.	Choose a source that contains vitamin E to prevent oxidation.
Potassium	See your healthcare provider for dosage instructions.	
Selenium	100 to 200 mcg once a day.	
Taurine	1.5 to 3 g once a day.	Consult with your healthcare provider before taking if you have liver or kidney disease.
Vitamin B complex	Use as directed.	
Vitamin C	500 mg twice a day.	Consult with your healthcare provider if you are prone to kidney stones or gout.
Vitamin D	Use as directed.	May cause poor appetite, nausea, and vomiting.
Vitamin E	200 to 400 IU once a day.	Take mixed tocopherols, the more active form of vitamin E. Consult with your health-care provider before taking if you are using a blood thinner.

HORMONE THERAPY

As you will see in Chapter 4, hormone balance is essential for helping you maintain memory and focus throughout your lifetime. Hormones also play an important role in regulating your cardiovascular system.

Accordingly, because your hormone levels decline as you age, you may want to consider hormone replacement therapy in order to protect both your cardiovascular system and your mind. When undertaken with a doctor's supervision, hormone replacement therapy can vastly improve your blood circulation and thus limit or prevent memory loss and cognitive decline. Below, you will find a discussion of various hormones that, when used properly, can have many benefits for preventing and treating heart diseases.

Estrogen

If estrogen therapy is initiated before the onset of menopause, it may have significant benefits in protecting against atherosclerosis in women. Estrogen has a number of other more general functions for heart health, some of which are listed below.

- Helps preserve your heart's ability to contract

- Helps prevent or limit the formation of plaque and calcium deposits, both of which contribute to the narrowing of the arteries.

- Helps repair wounds in blood vessels

- Improves the functioning of the arteries

- Improves insulin sensitivity

- Increases the volume of blood pumped by your heart

- Limits the development of atherosclerotic plaque and arterial calcification

- Lowers levels of fibrinogen, a substance that increases production of blood clots

- Suppresses the stress responses that can lead to high cholesterol, elevated blood sugar, high blood pressure, heart disease, and weight gain

Studies indicate that for postmenopausal women, estrogen replacement therapy may reduce the risk of heart disease and death due to heart disease by up to 50 percent. When used appropriately by postmenopausal women, estrogen can:

- Decrease total cholesterol

- Lower LDL (bad) cholesterol

- Raise HDL (good cholesterol)

- Improve blood pressure by acting as a calcium channel blocker and helping to keep blood vessels dilated (widened), allowing for better blood flow

In men, elevated levels of estrogen are associated with an increased risk of heart disease and prostate cancer. Furthermore, high levels of a specific type of estrogen, estradiol, are associated with an increased incidence of strokes, peripheral vascular disease, and carotid artery stenosis in men. Consequently, it is very important that men monitor their estrogen levels to detect any abnormalities.

Progesterone

In women, some evidence shows that progesterone, though not its synthetic equivalent progestin, enhances the benefits that estrogen exerts in preventing exercise-induced heart damage. Progesterone relaxes coronary arteries and helps prevent palpitations (the feeling you're your heart is racing or pounding). Progesterone has also been shown to lower blood pressure in women.

In men, progesterone replacement is a relatively recent treatment option. Studies show that progesterone replacement can lower triglycerides, total cholesterol, LDL (bad) cholesterol, apo B, and apo A-1—all markers that indicate higher risk of heart disease on a blood test.

Testosterone

Low testosterone levels are associated with cardiovascular conditions that increase the risk of memory decline, including diabetes, hypertension, and congestive heart failure.

In women who are testosterone deficient, hormone replacement therapy has the following benefits:

- Decreases symptoms of angina (chest pain)

- Lowers lipoprotein(a) levels by up to 65 percent

- Relaxes coronary arteries, allowing more blood to flow to the heart

Women whose estrogen levels are low should not undergo testosterone replacement, as this imbalance can increase your risk of heart disease. Thus, if you are considering testosterone replacement, you will also need to consider supplementing your estrogen and progesterone levels.

High testosterone levels in women are often a symptom of polycystic ovary syndrome (PCOS), a condition that is regularly associated with abnormal lipids and increased risk of heart disease, particularly hypertension. Accordingly, women with this condition should with a metabolic or anti-aging specialist who can help them lower their testosterone concentrations to a normal level.

In men, low testosterone levels are associated with cardiovascular conditions that increase the risk of memory decline, including diabetes, hypertension, and congestive heart failure. As men hit andropause, their testosterone levels begin to drop at a rate of one percent each year. This decrease in testosterone contributes to the elevated cholesterol levels often associated with the aging process. Therefore, to help prevent heart disease and maintain memory, men should consider testosterone replacement therapy if their levels are low.

DHEA-S

Low levels of dehydroepiandrosterone (DHEA-S) in men are associated with an increased risk of the development of heart disease. Likewise, low DHEA-S concentration has also been shown to be correlated with an increased risk of death from heart disease in men over the age of 50. In women, low DHEA-S levels have been associated with a higher rate of mortality from heart disease and also a higher rate of death from all causes.

Melatonin

Patients with coronary heart disease tend to have low nocturnal serum levels of melatonin. Melatonin has been shown to prevent damage in patients who have chronic oxygen deprivation due to the restriction of blood flow to the heart. Melatonin helps protect the heart by widening the blood vessels and attacking free radicals that damage your arteries; it is also known to inhibit the oxidation of LDL ("bad") cholesterol.

Thyroid Hormones

The link between dysfunction of the thyroid and cardiovascular disease has been known for more than a hundred years. Studies have shown that low thyroid function (hypothyroidism) is associated with an increased risk of heart disease. By optimizing your thyroid hormone levels, you can help keep your blood vessels flexible and dilated (widened), improve your lipid profile and insulin sensitivity, decrease your risk of congestive heart failure, and lower your levels of C-reactive protein and homocysteine—both substances associated with increased rates of heart disease. Consequently, it is important that your thyroid functions properly in order to prevent and treat heart disease. If you have questions about your thyroid function, see a metabolic or anti-aging specialist to help you measure your thyroid hormone levels.

Cortisol

The stress hormone cortisol plays an important role in heart health. In the INTERHEART study, a major international review of the risk factors that contribute to heart attack, psychosocial factors like stress were shown to be more potent predictors of the incidence of heart attack than diabetes, smoking, hypertension, and obesity. High cortisol levels, associated with a state of high stress, increase the risk of heart disease by elevating cholesterol and blood sugar levels. In addition, high cortisol levels may contribute to the development of high blood pressure, weight gain, and thyroid dysfunction. To lower your cortisol levels, take the appropriate measures to reduce the amount of stress in your life; a guide to stress management is included in the second part of this book.

CONCLUSION

Having read this chapter, you now know that memory loss can be caused by the poor blood circulation associated with cardiovascular disease. In fact, memory loss can even be considered to be a symptom of a heart condition. While you cannot always prevent heart disease, you can mitigate its effects or even reduce your risk of ever developing it through lifestyle changes, diet, supplements, and hormone replacement. Left untreated, poor circulation can lead to heart attack and stroke, and thus also vascular dementia. By improving your blood circulation, you will send vital aid not only to your heart, but also to your mind—dramatically reducing your risk for memory loss.

Is Your Memory Loss Caused by Heavy Metal Poisoning?

QUESTIONNAIRE

This test was designed to help you determine whether heavy metal poisoning might be affecting your memory and cognition. Read each question carefully and place a check mark in the box that best represents your answer.

	Yes	No	Unsure
1. Do you live in a building built before 1978?	☐	☐	☐
2. Do you or your children regularly handle old toys or furniture painted before 1976?	☐	☐	☐
3. Do you work in an occupation that that brings you into frequent contact with pipes and other metal hardware?	☐	☐	☐
4. Do you frequently come in contact with welding or smelting processes?	☐	☐	☐
5. Do you work in the mining or ore-processing industries?	☐	☐	☐
6. Do you use pesticides, fertilizers, or livestock feed that contains heavy metals?	☐	☐	☐
7. Do you work in an auto shop?	☐	☐	☐
8. Do you eat fish or shellfish more than twice each week?	☐	☐	☐
9. Do you use aluminum cookware or foil?	☐	☐	☐
10. Do your hobbies involve soldering, jewelry making, or pottery glazing?	☐	☐	☐

If you answered "yes" to any of these questions, your memory loss may be the result of heavy metal poisoning.

3

Heavy Metal Poisoning

Toxins—chemical elements that are poisonous to humans—can impair memory and cognition in a number of ways. As you will see in Chapter 5, any foreign substance that is introduced to your body can cause inflammation. Because localized inflammations (inflammations that affect specific organs or regions of your body) can affect or even spread to other parts of your body, toxins can thus be very damaging to your brain. In addition to their role in causing inflammation, these toxins can also directly influence memory and cognition by incurring oxidative stress, by inactivating the neurotransmitters which are essential for all brain processes, and/or by damaging or interfering with the proper function of your nerves and brain cells.

While there are many toxins that can potentially harm your body, this chapter focuses on heavy metals—specific metals and metal compounds that can seriously affect your health. Heavy metals can inflict damage on many different organs and organ systems, including your heart, kidneys, bones, and immune system. But studies consistently show that heavy metals most commonly attack the nervous system, making them particularly hazardous to your brain and cognitive ability. What's troubling is that exposure to these metals is not limited to those who work in manufacturing or construction industries. In fact, you can be exposed to many harmful metals through the environment (soil, food, water), or through common consumer products (paint and other art materials, cosmetics, toys, dental work).

Most often, exposure occurs when you repeatedly come into contact with a metal over a long period of time; symptoms don't appear until significant amounts of the toxin accumulate in your system. This is called chronic metal poisoning. More rarely, acute metal poisoning occurs when you either ingest or are exposed to very large amounts of a toxin in a short period of time.

The questionnaire at the beginning of this chapter is designed to help you determine whether toxins are affecting your memory and focus. If you answered "yes" to any of the questions, you may be suffering from heavy metal poisoning. This chapter offers a general overview of heavy metal poisoning, providing you with a guide to understanding its primary sources, symptoms, diagnosis, and treatment methods. Armed with this information, you will be able to end or reduce your exposure to heavy metals, and thus remove a dangerous obstacle to your cognitive health.

SYMPTOMS

While the precise symptoms depend on the exact nature of the metal to which the victim is exposed, there are certain common physical and neurological markers that can indicate that chronic heavy metal poisoning has occurred. Besides memory loss, they include:

- Abdominal pain
- Blindness and vision problems
- Confusion
- Difficulty learning
- Gastrointestinal distress
- Loss of appetite

- Mood disorders
- Muscle weakness
- Rashes and other skin problems
- Seizures
- Speech problems
- Tremors

Unfortunately, it can be difficult to detect chronic exposure to heavy metals, as it takes time for the toxins to build up in your body and cause symptoms. Often, mild warning signs are ignored or mistaken for symptoms of other health problems; not until symptoms become worse is heavy metal poisoning suspected.

By contrast, it's relatively easy to recognize cases of acute heavy metal poisoning. Acute poisoning is very serious, and can potentially cause shock, kidney failure, and even death. Those who survive incidents of acute poisoning will experience symptoms of chronic poisoning as the toxin exits the body over time.

SOURCES

There are many different metals that act as toxins and can induce heavy metal poisoning. This section outlines the substances whose effects on cognition are best known.

Aluminum

Aluminum is a metal that is often found in food additives, car exhaust, tobacco smoke, foil, cans, ceramics, antacids, antidiarrheal medications, and in some food additives, antiperspirants, and infant immunizations. Prolonged or intensive exposure to aluminum has been shown by some studies to be associated with nerve damage and the formation of amyloid plaques in the brain. As you'll recall from Chapter 1, amyloid plaques are themselves associated with the development of Alzheimer's disease and other forms of dementia; the more extensive the plaque growth, the greater the interference with your basic cognitive function.

Arsenic

Arsenic is a poison that can be found in small quantities in certain pesticides, drugs, microelectronics, car exhaust, and chemical weapons. Chronic exposure to arsenic can occur in those who work in various mining and manufacturing industries, car repair, or in those who are engaged in gardening and agriculture (due to the use of arsenic in pesticides, livestock feed, and cotton harvesting). Outside of occupational exposure, arsenic poisoning can arise from tainted well water or soil; arsenic can also be found in certain food additives (including apple juice) and in phosphate detergents. Prolonged or intensive exposure to arsenic can cause extensive damage to the peripheral nervous system, as a result, learning, recent memory, and concentration are all impaired. Arsenic may also interfere with the proper functioning of a gene that helps produce and regulate insulin, increasing the likelihood of diabetes, which is a significant risk factor in and of itself for decreased focus and memory.

Copper

When obtained in appropriate amounts, the micromineral copper is actually essential for the health of your brain, functioning as an antioxidant and helping to protect against free radical damage. Most people receive all the copper they need through diet—seafood, organ meats (liver, kidneys), whole grains, legumes (beans), and nuts are particularly rich in this nutrient.

Because copper is critical to the maintenance of your brain's bio-chemistry, copper levels that are too high or too low can result in neurological disorders. Overexposure to copper can occur in those who work in welding or the manufacture of microelectronics and batteries; other sources of occupational exposure include certain paints, insecticides and fungicides, ceramics, artificial flowers, fabric dyes, rayon, and wood preservatives. High copper levels are associated with the accumulation of amyloid plaques and tau tangles, both hallmarks of Alzheimer's disease (see pages 101 and 104).

Fluoride

While not technically a heavy metal, fluoride is a chemical element that is frequently added to local water sources and toothpaste due to its benefits in preventing tooth decay. It can also be found in some fruit juices, soft drinks, and infant foods. Studies in China have shown that children living in areas where water is fluoridated tend to have IQs that are ten to twenty points lower than those of children living in low-fluoride areas. Furthermore, animal studies have shown that fluoride can cross the blood-brain barrier and instigate short-term memory loss. More studies need to be done concerning fluoride exposure and cognitive function in humans.

Iron

Iron is a micromineral that plays many important roles in maintaining your body's health. Perhaps most notably, iron is a key ingredient in your red blood cells, allowing for the transport of oxygen throughout your circulatory system. Ideally, you would get all the iron you need through your diet; natural sources include kelp, many whole grains and seeds, red meat, and leafy greens like beet greens and Swiss chard. While iron deficiency is common and can contribute to memory loss, overexposure to iron can be much more serious, at least where your brain is concerned. High levels of iron are associated with an accelerated rate of accumulation of amyloid plaques, a hallmark of Alzheimer's disease. Elevated iron levels also seem to be implicated in the brain inflammation that often accompanies Alzheimer's disease, impairing the immune response to oxidative stress and free radical damage. Iron poisoning is rare, but can be caused by overconsumption of iron supplements.

Lead

The National Institutes of Health consider lead to be a "very strong poison" that can lead to serious health problems. Although campaigns to raise awareness of the dangers of lead poisoning have been successful in many regards—gasoline and house paint are no longer manufactured with this substance—lead can still be found in old homes; toys painted before 1976 or outside the United States; certain art supplies; pottery, pewter dinnerware; and older plumbing, pipes, and metal fixtures. Lead can also be found in dirt and dust that has been contaminated by old car exhaust, paint chips, or metal residues. Outside of the domestic sphere, lead poisoning can be occupational, resulting from exposure due to participation in various types of manufacturing and mining enterprises.

Although lead can affect every organ in your body, lead's primary target is the nervous system. Over time, lead can accumulate in your body, leading to brain damage. Lead poisoning is especially serious for children; exposure can prevent proper brain development and lead to lifelong learning disabilities, behavioral problems, and speech disorders. In adults, long-term exposure can lead to serious cognitive decline, including memory loss, impaired concentration, and mood disorders. Even low-level lead exposure has been associated with cognitive decline.

While lead can directly cause the death or dysfunction of neurons and other nerve cells, it can also affect cognition indirectly. High concentrations of lead are associated with increased levels of homocysteine, an amino acid that promotes free radical production. As you will see in Chapter 5, free radicals are unstable molecules that wreak havoc on your body's cells, damaging or killing them as part of the inflammatory process called oxidative stress. High lead levels also contribute to high blood pressure, itself a risk factor for vascular dementia and other circulation-related memory loss.

Manganese

Manganese is a mineral that can be found naturally in many nuts, seeds, and grains. When possessed in appropriate concentrations, manganese actually plays a number of important roles in your body. It helps the body manufacture connective tissue, bones, and sex hormones, and is involved in carbohydrate metabolism, calcium absorption, and blood sugar regulation. It also acts as an antioxidant, protecting the body against damage by free radicals. Perhaps most important to our discussion, manganese is also considered to be essential for proper brain and nerve function.

Moderate levels of manganese are thus beneficial to your body. The trouble starts when manganese levels exceed the accepted limits. For most people, manganese toxicity is not an issue, or even a possibility; normal levels of manganese are maintained through diet and outside exposure is unlikely. Manganese toxicity is a risk, however, for those who endure occupational exposure to manganese. People who weld or smelt as part of a manufacturing industry, or who come into prolonged contact with manganese through contaminated drinking water or the use of certain fertilizers or art supplies, are likely to inhale manganese, which then travels directly to the brain, where it can inflict serious damage to neurons. High brain levels of manganese are associated with neurological problems such as tremors, mood changes, and hallucinations; and disorders such as Parkinson's disease—itself a potential cause of dementia (see Chapter 1). Chronic manganese exposure may also impair brain development in children, causing poor cognitive performance.

Mercury

Chronic mercury exposure and inhalation can cause serious neurological damage, leading to cognitive decline, psychological issues, and mood disorders. Mercury poisoning is particularly dangerous to children, in whom mercury can impede development and potentially cause learning disabilities and even mental retardation. It does this by interfering with the production of antioxidants, essentially causing oxidative stress (see page 73), which in turn leads to the degeneration of neurons. Toxic levels of mercury also throw your neurotransmitter levels out of balance, endangering proper communication between your brain cells. In addition, mercury may also increase the production of neurofibrillary tangles and amyloid proteins—both brain hallmarks of various forms of dementia, including Alzheimer's disease. (See Chapter 1).

Remember the Mad Hatter in *Alice in Wonderland*? The concept of the mad hatter is rooted in fact: many eighteenth- and nineteenth-century milliners developed emotional disturbances and dementia due to their constant contact with mercury, which was used to produce and treat the felt used in hatmaking. While mercury is no longer used to manufacture hats, it can be found in certain thermometers, electrical and medical equipment, older dental fillings, and some disinfectants.

Mercury is also emitted into the air by power plants and some facilities engaged in industrial manufacturing. From the air, it can make its way into various bodies of water, where it is transformed by naturally-occurring bacteria into methyl mercury, a form of mercury that is particularly dangerous to humans. Fish living in these bodies of water can accumulate higher levels of methyl mercury; when you eat these fish on a regular basis, you can put yourself at risk for mercury poisoning. Although the Environmental Protection Agency (EPA) claims that nearly all fish and shellfish contain at least traces of methyl mercury, larger fishes tend to have higher levels, since they have had more time to grow, and thus also more time to accumulate dangerous amounts of this harmful metal. For this reason, the EPA recommends limiting your intake of even low-mercury fish (shrimp, canned light tuna, pollock, and catfish) to twelve ounces a week and avoiding shark, swordfish, king mackerel, and tilefish altogether. Because mercury poisoning develops gradually, you don't have to be too strict about this weekly recommendation; if you eat fish more than twice in one week, simply scale back your fish consumption the following week.

Zinc

Zinc is an important micromineral that is used in over a hundred enzymatic reactions in your body. Most people get all the zinc they need through their diet; food sources rich in zinc include oysters and other seafood, red meat, fresh ginger, beans, and nuts. Like any nutrient, however, too much of this mineral can be toxic to the body, especially the brain; elevated levels of zinc increase the rate at which amyloid plaques are formed. Overexposure can occur occupationally to those in manufacturing industries, or to those who routinely come into zinc through work with automotive components, electrical equipment, tools, hardware, and certain toys.

DIAGNOSIS

Because heavy metal poisoning is rare, it can sometimes be mistaken for other illnesses or disorders. Often, heavy metal poisoning will be considered as a diagnosis simply by dint of patient history and current lifestyle factors. If you are engaged in an occupation or lifestyle that brings you into repeated contact with a metal or metals, for example, you are more likely to be at risk for heavy metal poisoning. Without a clear source of contamination, diagnosis can only be confirmed with certain tests, which vary depending on the toxin suspected to be causing symptoms; blood and urine tests are most commonly used to determine whether metal levels are high. If you suspect heavy metal poisoning has occurred, consult with your healthcare provider and request that testing to be done.

PREVENTION

With heavy metal poisoning, prevention is often the best treatment. Now that you are aware of the dangers of heavy metal toxicity, it is time to reduce or eliminate its presence in your life. The following tips will help you to identify and get rid of any heavy metals you might come into contact with on a regular basis:

- Scrape or seal off rooms painted before 1978. Painting over old paint will not eliminate the lead contained within. Because the very process of paint removal can be hazardous to your health, if you suspect that your rooms have old paint layers, consult a professional to get the toxins removed.

- Avoid giving children old toys to play with. Toys made before 1976 may be decorated with leaded paint.

- Don't use aluminum cookware, and limit your use of aluminum foil.

- If you have mercury fillings, consider having an environmental dentist replace them with direct composite, porcelain, or gold fillings.

- Limit your consumption of fish and shellfish to species that are low in mercury, such as sardines, tilapia, shrimp, and oysters.

- Throw out household detergents, pesticides, fertilizers, and art supplies that contain heavy metals—read the ingredient lists to see whether aluminum, arsenic, manganese or phosphates are included. Instead, use green household products, which are less toxic and thus safe for domestic use.

- If your job puts you in close proximity to heavy metals, make sure you take the appropriate measures to avoid contamination. Wear goggles, a mask, and/or gloves when needed. The Occupational Safety and Health Administration (OSHA) publishes strict rules for industries that use heavy metals in their manufacturing. To make sure your workplace follows these rules, look for more information on OSHA's website, www.osha.gov.

p 38 - negative effects of flouride

testosterone level

strength ex.

word lists - cards played

Ron

groups.

bananas at bedtime.

...to transfer your annuity assets, a surrender or liquidation of your annuity contract assets must generally occur. This may result in the following consequences: surrender charges, loss of vested living or death benefits, taxable earnings and possible tax penalties. For annuities not held in an IRA account, Section 1035 of the Internal Revenue Code allows you to make a tax-free exchange of one annuity contract for another annuity contract. Some annuities require the submission of the original policy to complete a transfer; please consult with your Insurance Company and submit the original policy if needed.

How do I transfer my company retirement plans?

Please consult with your plan administrator before initiating a transfer request. Then, to roll over your 401(k) or another employer-sponsored retirement plan, call a Schwab Rollover Consultant at **1-877-412-6116.** From filling out paperwork to answering your questions and helping you work with your plan administrator, a dedicated Rollover Consultant will personally manage the process for you from start to finish, making it easy to roll over to a new IRA.

What about cost basis?

Schwab will update your account with the cost basis information provided on a transfer statement by a delivering firm. Because the accuracy of cost basis data depends upon these third-party statements, Schwab is not able to guarantee the availability, accuracy or completeness of such cost basis data. It is your obligation to confirm the accuracy of the information Schwab receives from the delivering firm by visiting www.schwab.com or calling Schwab. Cost basis information is intended for residents of the U.S. It may not be available or appropriate for customers who reside outside the U.S.

Questions? Call 1-800-435-4000.
Thank you for investing with Charles Schwab.

...However, some may take up to six weeks

Please remember that while we make every effort to ensure a swift transfer, the actual transfer time depends on how quickly securities are liquidated and released or transferred by the financial institution currently holding your investments.

Will I be charged a fee?

An exit fee may be charged by your previous financial institution upon receiving your transfer request. A wire fee may also be charged by your previous financial institution to transfer to Schwab.

Fractional shares of stock are nontransferable, and any fractional shares will be liquidated by the delivering firm upon the transfer of the whole shares. The delivering firm may or may not charge a fee for this liquidation.

If the assets you are transferring are considered nonstandard assets at Schwab (such as limited partnerships), there will be set-up and maintenance fees.

Are my funds transferable?

Schwab can transfer over 6,000 different mutual funds. Some financial firms issue their own (proprietary) mutual funds, and these funds typically cannot be transferred to any firm. Also, there are some mutual fund companies with whom Schwab has not established an agreement with the fund issuer to hold a particular mutual fund. If the mutual fund cannot be transferred, then you may be notified by mail.

How do I sell assets prior to transfer?

If there are assets that need to be sold before being transferred to Schwab, please instruct the delivering firm to sell assets in your brokerage or trust company account and cancel dividend reinvestment **prior**

TREATMENT OPTIONS

In the event that heavy metal poisoning is diagnosed, the first order of business will be to address the source of the problem. If possible, reduce or eliminate your exposure to any toxic substances, as discussed above: remove lead from your environment by getting rid of (or sealing off) old paint and throwing out toys made before the eighties, stop using aluminum foil and aluminum-based antiperspirants, and limit your consumption of fish containing high levels of mercury.

Chronic heavy metal poisoning may require chelation therapy. Chelation therapy involves the injection or ingestion of a chemical—most often ethylenediaminetetraacetic acid (EDTA) or dimercaptosuccinic acid (DMSA)—that will bind to (chelate) heavy metals, including lead, mercury, and arsenic. Once these toxic metals have been attached to the chemical binder, they can then be removed from your system through urination. Typically, chelation therapy involves between five and thirty treatments; each session can last up to several hours if the chelating agent is delivered by an IV line. Depending on the type and severity of the poisoning, treatment can take several months to complete; recovery is slow and gradual. Possible side effects include fever, nausea, vomiting, low blood pressure, and headache. Because chelation therapy binds indiscriminately to all metals and minerals in your body, your doctor will likely prescribe supplements that replace the nutrients that are stripped from your body.

Acute cases of metal poisoning require immediate emergency treatment. If you have ingested a large amount of a toxin, you will need to empty your stomach within four hours of the incident; if not, emergency medical technicians will likely administer antidotes designed to inactivate the dangerous metals. Those who survive acute heavy metal poisoning may still need to undergo chelation therapy in order to eliminate the remaining toxins.

CONCLUSION

Although heavy metal poisoning is rare, its effects on your brain and nervous system can be extensive and wide-ranging, leading to cognitive decline and memory loss. As you will see in Chapter 5, one of the most important things you can do for your mind is to prevent harmful substances from entering your body. Toxins such as heavy metals must be avoided if at all possible in order to ensure that your mind is sharp and active for years to come.

Is Your Memory Loss Caused by Hormonal Imbalance?

This test was designed to help you determine whether a hormonal imbalance might be affecting your memory and cognition. Read each question carefully and place a check mark in the box that best represents your answer.

	Yes	No	Unsure
1. Are you under a lot of stress?	☐	☐	☐
2. Are you taking any pharmaceutical drugs, such as antibiotics, antidepressants, birth control pills, or painkillers?	☐	☐	☐
3. Are you overweight by twenty pounds or more?	☐	☐	☐
4. Do you exercise infrequently?	☐	☐	☐
5. Do you suffer from an endocrine disorder (disease of the pituitary, thyroid, parathyroid, adrenal, and pancreatic glands)?	☐	☐	☐
6. Are you currently undergoing chemotherapy?	☐	☐	☐

For Women:

	Yes	No	Unsure
7. Are you currently experiencing menopause or perimenopause?	☐	☐	☐
8. Do you suffer from endometriosis, premature ovarian decline, or polycystic ovary syndrome (PCOS)?	☐	☐	☐
9. Are you pregnant?	☐	☐	☐

For Men:

	Yes	No	Unsure
10. Are you over fifty and currently experiencing andropause (male menopause?)	☐	☐	☐

If you answered "yes" to any of these questions, your memory loss may be the result of a hormonal imbalance.

4

Hormonal Imbalance

Memory loss can be a symptom of hormonal imbalance. Hormones are the chemical messengers of your body; they travel through your bloodstream delivering signals that tell your cells to carry out many of the tasks that are essential for your survival. While they are best known for regulating a wide variety of important processes—including sexual function, reproduction, metabolism, and growth—hormones also play an important role in maintaining proper cognitive function and memory.

Your hormones are in constant communication, each one performing a specific part in your body's hormonal symphony. In order for your mind and body to function properly, your hormones must work in harmony. When your hormones are balanced, the symphony plays in tune; you feel great and your mind spins along at maximum speed. When your hormones are not balanced, the symphony plays out of tune; you feel lousy and you have difficulty remembering things or executing simple mental tasks.

Thus, if you or a loved one suffer from memory loss, it could very well be the result of a hormonal imbalance or dysfunction (overproduction or underproduction of a hormone). The questionnaire at the beginning of this chapter is designed to help you determine whether this is the case. If you answered "yes" to many of the questions above, it is possible that a hormonal imbalance is impairing your cognitive ability. This chapter will provide you with valuable information about the causes and symptoms of hormonal imbalance, the roles played by specific hormones in supporting memory and cognitive function, and what you can do to resolve any deficiencies or excesses you might have.

First, let's look at the reasons hormonal imbalances occur.

CAUSES OF HORMONAL IMBALANCES

There are many factors that influence the amounts of hormones your body produces, and the way they balance out. While your hormone levels generally decrease as you age, it's important to understand that hormonal dysfunction is not simply a problem suffered by seniors and the middle-aged—young people can be affected, too! Throughout your lifetime, your hormone levels are constantly changing, fluctuating from hour to hour, day to day, and year to year. Here, we are concerned solely with factors that have long-term effects for your hormonal balance, as these are the factors that are most likely to also affect your memory and cognition. Although the specific cause of a hormonal imbalance or dysfunction will depend on your personal situation and the hormone affected, the following is a list of general factors that can cause hormone problems.

Causes of Hormonal Imbalances

- Alcohol abuse

- Andropause (male menopause)

- Caffeine

- Chemotherapy

- Childbirth

- Endocrine disorders (diseases of the pituitary, thyroid, parathyroid, adrenal, and pancreatic glands)

- Endometriosis

- Environmental toxins

- Genetics

- Head injury

- Infection

- Lack of exercise or too much exercise

- Nutritional deficiencies

- Obesity

- Certain pharmaceutical drugs (including antidepressants, birth control pills, etc.)

- Perimenopause and menopause

- Polycystic ovary syndrome (PCOS)

- Poor diet (diet low in grains and fiber, high in saturated fats and sugar)

- Pregnancy

- Recreational drug use

- Stress

- Vitamin deficiencies

PREGNENOLONE

Pregnenolone is a neurosteroid hormone—that is, a hormone that primarily affects the functioning of your brain cells (neurons). It is made by both your brain and the adrenal glands. Pregnenolone is often called the "mother hormone" because it is used to produce many other important hormones, including cortisol, DHEA, estrogen, progesterone, and testosterone. Besides its role in producing other hormones, pregnenolone has many functions: it helps regulate and repair your nervous system, increases energy, boosts resistance to stress, guards against insomnia, and reduces pain and inflammation. But above all, pregnenolone has significant influence over your memory. Pregnenolone is essential to the functioning of your brain cells: it helps supply them with energy, increases their resistance to stress, and repairs nerve damage. It also enhances your brain cells' capacity to convey messages by regulating certain neurotransmitters and neurotransmitter receptors.

Pregnenolone levels naturally decrease with age—by age seventy-five, you are likely to have 65 percent less pregnenolone than you do at thirty-five. Because pregnenolone is essential for cognitive function, and because it also plays such an integral role in the synthesis of other hormones that affect memory, it is important to make sure you achieve the appropriate level of this important hormone. Some studies show that by supplementing your pregnenolone levels, you can improve your memory and cognitive performance.

Symptoms of Pregnenolone Deficiency

- Arthritis
- Depression
- Fatigue

- Inability to deal with stress
- Insomnia
- Lack of focus/cognitive decline

ESTROGEN

Estrogen is a general term for a group of "female" sex hormones—so called because they are primarily associated with a woman's ability to conceive and bear children. But estrogen's influence is not limited to reproduction. Although estrogen is made primarily in a woman's ovaries, receptor sites for this important hormone can be found in a woman's brain, muscles, bones, bladder, gut, uterus, vagina, breasts, eyes, heart, lungs, and blood vessels. Accordingly, estrogen has been shown to have over 400 different functions in a woman's body. It helps regulate body temperature and blood pressure, prevents muscle damage, improves mood, and increases libido. In addition, it is believed to increase metabolism, maintain skin and artery elasticity, and help optimize cholesterol levels.

It's important to note that while estrogen is seen as a "female" hormone, it is also produced and used by men. In men, estrogen primarily helps to preserve bone structure and is involved in lipid (fat) metabolism.

Function in Memory and Cognition

Estrogen also plays an important role in regulating brain function, and thus memory loss. As Dr. Frederick Naftolin, director of reproductive

Estrogen and the Female Brain

Estrogen is a powerful hormone that can exert enormous influence on the female brain. Estrogen can actually alter the neurochemistry and structure of the brain in ways that improve cognition. Among other functions, estrogen:

• Coordinates the healing and regrowth of nerve cells in response to strokes and other brain damage

• Helps maintain and increase nerve connectivity and complexity in the brain

• Increases the surface area of potential "docking sites" on neurons for incoming messages

• Boosts the metabolism of the brain by promoting its uptake of glucose, its basic energy source

• Protects your nerve cells from damage by acting as an anti-inflammatory, boosting the body's natural antioxidants (which fight free radicals), and guarding against plaque deposits

• Reduces the formation of amyloid plaques, the toxic brain-destroying protein deposits implicated in Alzheimer's disease

biology research at the New York University Langone Medical Center, has asserted, "there is not a cell in the brain that is not directly or indirectly sensitive to estrogen." The processes of thinking, remembering, and focusing all rely heavily on estrogen as a "transmission fluid" that helps conduct and project messages through the major areas of your brain, especially the hippocampus.

Women produce three main types of estrogen: estrone (E1), estradiol (E2), and estriol (E3). During menopause, levels of estradiol—the strongest form of estrogen, and the one most responsible for maintaining brain function—begin to drop. Estradiol levels can also decrease if you have had one or both of your ovaries removed before menopause. Lack of this hormone can be problematic; research shows that lower estradiol levels are associated with memory loss. As a result, many doctors have recommended estrogen replacement therapy. When taken as directed,

---

• Stimulates the production of various neurotransmitters that are heavily involved in cognitive and memory processes, including acetylcholine, dopamine, gamma-aminobutyric acid (GABA), glutamate, noradrenaline, and serotonin

As a result, when administered as part of a hormone replacement therapy at the onset of menopause, estrogen can have the following effects:

• Acts as an upper, increasing energy and feelings of wellbeing

• Boosts metabolic activity of many areas of the brain and spinal cord within hours of administration

• Decreases distractibility

• Increases manual speed and dexterity in women

• Increases performance and speed of learning on sensory-motor tasks

• Increases sensory perception: hearing, smell, visual signal detection, ad fine touch

• Increases short-term memory

• Increases verbal fluency, speech ability, articulation agility, syllable repetition, speeded counting, and word reading

• Maintains central processing motor integration in tasks such as driving

estrogen has been shown to increase cerebral circulation and reduce the likelihood of developing Alzheimer's disease by as much as 54 percent. For specific areas of cognition that see improvement after estrogen therapy, see the inset on page 49.

Estrogen is known to help maintain memory in men, too; it acts as a neuroprotector, guarding men's brain cells against damage and death. Perhaps for this reason, low levels of estrogen are seen alongside low testosterone levels in men with Alzheimer's disease. Estrogen replacement therapy is generally not necessary for men, since low levels are rare.

Symptoms of Estrogen Deficiency (Women)

- Abdominal weight gain
- Acne
- Anxiety
- Arthritis
- Chronic fatigue syndrome
- Decrease in sexual interest/ function
- Depression
- Diabetes
- Difficulty losing weight, even with diet and exercise
- Elevated blood pressure
- Elevated cholesterol

- Food cravings
- Increase in headaches and migraines
- Increase in facial hair
- Infertility
- Joint pain
- Low energy
- Osteoporosis/osteopenia
- Polycystic ovary syndrome
- Restless sleep
- Thinner skin
- Vaginal dryness or pain

Symptoms of Estrogen Deficiency (Men)

- Osteoporosis/osteopenia

PROGESTERONE

Progesterone is a sex hormone and neurosteroid that is made in the ovaries of premenopausal women and in the adrenal glands of postmenopausal women, and in the testicular tissue and adrenal glands of men. In women, progesterone balances estrogen, playing a role in menstruation, pregnancy, and the formation of embryos. It is also involved in sleep patterns, bone development, bladder function, and mood. In men, progesterone primarily influences the generation of sperm and the production of testosterone. Progesterone in males may also regulate blood sugar, decrease the risk of prostate cancer, and help with depression.

Function in Memory and Cognition

In both sexes, progesterone has many positive effects on neurons. It helps regulate brain levels of certain neurotransmitters associated with learning and memory, including dopamine and GABA.

Scientists are now looking at progesterone replacement to aid in the prevention of memory loss. One study found that progesterone treatment reduced the impairment in spatial, reference, and working memory in patients who had suffered global cerebral ischemia, a condition in which the brain does not receive enough oxygen as the result of a heart attack or stroke. In addition, progesterone was found to prevent the narrowing of the brain's memory center, the hippocampus, which is otherwise damaged by ischemia.

Symptoms of Progesterone Deficiency (Women)

- Anxiety
- Decreased HDL levels
- Decreased libido
- Depression
- Excessive or heavy menstruation
- Hypersensitivity
- Insomnia
- Irritability
- Migraine headaches prior to menstrual cycles
- Mood swings
- Nervousness
- Osteoporosis
- Pain and inflammation
- Weight gain

Because there is relatively little research on the role of progesterone in men, medical science has not yet established the definitive symptoms associated with male progesterone deficiency.

TESTOSTERONE

Testosterone falls into a class of hormones called androgens, or "male" hormones—so called because these hormones tend to control human functions and characteristics that are considered to be male. In men, testosterone is made in the testicles, and regulates the formation of male reproductive organs. In women, testosterone is made in the adrenal glands and ovaries, and is associated with improving libido, bone density, muscle tone, mood, and energy levels.

In both men and women, testosterone levels decrease with age. This decline is more pronounced in men. After the age of thirty, men's testosterone levels can fall at a rate of approximately 1 percent each year. By their seventies, 30 to 60 percent of all men are hypogonadal, meaning that they have lost some hormonal function. The time in a man's life when he is losing hormonal balance is called andropause.

Function in Memory and Cognition

Testosterone is important to cognition in both men and women. In fact, the development of memory loss in men may be directly related to the loss of testosterone that occurs as a result of age. In men, low levels of testosterone are consistently shown to be associated with various levels of memory loss, including Alzheimer's disease. Studies show that low testosterone levels may affect many different types of memory, including visual and verbal memory, and spatial and mathematical reasoning. In general, the lower a man's testosterone level, the greater his risk of developing some form of memory loss. Scientists believe that this is because the depletion of testosterone leads to increased brain cell (neuron) death, higher antibody levels, increased production of the amyloid-B proteins associated with Alzheimer's disease and other forms of dementia. Conversely, higher levels of testosterone are associated with better performance in specific aspects of memory and cognitive function, including spatial cognition, verbal fluency, and working memory.

Testosterone replacement in men has been shown to improve verbal and spatial memory, and even to help reverse some cognitive dysfunction. Studies have suggested testosterone therapy can also protect against Alzheimer's disease by helping to prevent the production of amyloid-B protein (see Chapter 7). In addition, testosterone replacement has been shown to decrease men's risk of developing cardiovascular disease, itself an independent risk factor for cognitive decline (see Chapter 2).

There's evidence that testosterone replacement can also help women's cognition. Recently, a small pilot study showed that testosterone therapy can help protect the memory of healthy aging women. Another study indicated that testosterone treatment improved verbal learning and memory in postmenopausal women.

Symptoms of Testosterone Deficiency (Men)

- Fatigue, tiredness, or loss of energy
- Depression, low or negative mood
- Irritability, anger, or bad temper
- Anxiety or nervousness
- Loss of concentration
- Loss of sexual drive or libido
- Loss of erections or other problems during sex
- Decreased intensity of orgasms
- Backache, joint pains or stiffness
- Loss of fitness
- Feeling overstressed
- Decrease in job performance
- Decline in physical abilities
- Osteopenia/osteoporosis (bone loss)
- Elevated cholesterol

Symptoms of Testosterone Deficiency (Women)

- Anxiety
- Decline in muscle tone
- Decreased HDL (good cholesterol)
- Decreased sex drive
- Droopy eyelids
- Dry, thin skin and hair
- Fatigue
- Hypersensitive, hyperemotional states
- Less dreaming
- Loss of pubic hair
- Low self-esteem
- Mild depression
- Muscle wasting (despite adequate calorie and protein intake)
- Saggy cheeks
- Weight gain

DHEA

Dehydroepiandrosterone (DHEA) is a neurosteroid hormone that is produced by the adrenal glands. DHEA is the precursor to male and female sex hormones, meaning that it can be converted into estrogen and testosterone. The primary function of DHEA is to balance the stress hormone cortisol, but it also seems to play roles in weight loss and cardiovascular health.

DHEA production naturally declines with age, with levels starting to drop for both men and women in the late twenties. By age seventy, your body makes only a quarter of the DHEA it once made during peak production. As a result, it is unlikely that your body will ever produce too much DHEA. If your DHEA levels are high, it is probably the result of an improperly calibrated hormone replacement therapy.

Function in Memory and Cognition

Low DHEA levels are often caused by stress and the aging process, and can lead to cognitive decline. In one study, researchers found that patients with Alzheimer's disease had DHEA levels that were 48 percent lower than those of their normal counterparts. Medical studies are mixed as to whether DHEA replacement has a strong effect on memory, but some evidence suggests that it might. A recent double-blind, placebo-controlled, crossover study in which DHEA was given to post-menopausal women showed that DHEA replacement therapy improved performance ona variety of visual and spatial tasks, including mental rotation, subject-ordered pointing, fragmented picture identification, perceptual identification, and same-different judgment.

Symptoms of DHEA Deficiency

- Decreased energy
- Decreased muscle strength
- Difficulty dealing with stress

- Increased risk of infection
- Irritability
- Joint soreness
- Weight gain

CORTISOL

Cortisol is the main steroid hormone produced by your adrenal glands. Cortisolis best known as your primary stress hormone. Stress hormones play an integral role in protecting us from perceived threats. When you find yourself in a situation that your brain interprets as dangerous—say, you're approached by a man with a gun—your body releases stress hormones like cortisol in order to help you cope. Cortisol performs a number of different tasks: first, it suppresses any bodily functions that are not essential to helping you deal with the situation: your digestion, reproductive capacity, immune function, and growth processes. Then, it temporarily boosts your energy levels by both increasing the availability of sugar (glucose) in your bloodstream and enhancing the ability of your brain and muscles to use that sugar. As a result, your body is better equipped to either combat the threat or escape it—a choice scientists call the "fight-or-flight" response. Once the threat has been dispatched, cortisol leaves your system and your body goes back to the way it was before you encountered the dangerous situation.

The "fight-or-flight" response is a built-in part of our bodies' evolutionary design, triggered not just by acute or short-term episodes of perceived danger, but by any situation we interpret as stressful—whether it's being chased by a gun-wielding robber or trying to pay off a large credit card bill. When deployed occasionally, your stress response is actually constructive, allowing you to deal successfully with perilous situations. But, as you'll see, in situations of chronic stress, your cortisol levels remain elevated for long periods of time, with harmful consequences.

Function in Memory and Cognition

When produced in normal amounts, cortisol is very useful for the maintenance of memory and brain function. In particular, cortisol helps to regulate the prefrontal cortex, the area of the brain that is responsible for working memory, personality expression, and critical analysis and decision-making.

Different factors can elevate your cortisol levels. Cortisol is the only hormone in your body whose levels actually increase as you age. As discussed above, stress can also increase the amount of cortisol your body produces. When you are under chronic or long-term stress, your body churns out more and more cortisol in an ongoing attempt to manage the pressure. This elevation in cortisol levels creates a number of negative consequences for your memory. Studies show that excess cortisol can destroy existing nerve cells and even rewire the electrical circuits of the brain. It can also indirectly cause the destruction of brain cells by stimu-

Chronic Stress and Adrenal Fatigue

Chronic stress is a pervasive problem in modern society, and one whose debilitating effects extend to many different aspects of individual health. If not properly treated, chronic stress can contribute not only to mental and mood dysfunction, but also to sleep disorders, cardiovascular disease, and even weight gain. Another potential outcome of chronic stress is a condition called adrenal fatigue, or hypocortisolism. Adrenal fatigue occurs when chronic stress has forced your levels of cortisol to remain elevated for a particularly long period of time. Exhausted from having to keep churning out stress hormones, your adrenal glands simply give up or "burn out." When this happens, your cortisol and DHEA levels drop dramatically. You feel tired and unwell, and you may have trouble thinking and concentrating. Because these low cortisol levels are essentially the result of chronic stress (prolonged high cortisol), treatment for adrenal fatigue involves stress management, as discussed here and in Chapter 11.

lating the production of free radicals, which inflict further damage. The hippocampus, your brain's memory center, is especially vulnerable to stress; when exposed to excess levels of cortisol, cells in the hippocampus begin to die. Damage to the hippocampus as the result of stress can also lead to memory loss, as a smaller or atrophied hippocampus is often seen in patients who suffer major depression, an independent risk factor for the onset of cognitive decline. As a result, high cortisol levels are associated with decreased cognitive function and increased risk of Alzheimer's disease and other forms of dementia and memory loss.

There is a simple solution that will allow you to prevent or reduce high cortisol levels: limit or eliminate the stress in your life! By restricting the amount of stress you are exposed to, you can make sure that your cortisol levels remain normal, thus guarding against a major source of memory loss. In Chapter 11, we discuss many of the techniques that you can use to guard against the excess cortisol levels associated with stress.

Symptoms of Excess Cortisol

- Binge eating
- Confusion
- Depression
- Fatigue

- Hypothyroidism (low thyroid function)

- Increased blood pressure

- Increased blood sugar/increased insulin

- Increased cholesterol

- Increased susceptibility to bruising

- Increased susceptibility to infections

- Increased triglycerides

- Irritability

- Low energy

- Memory loss

- Night sweats

- Osteopenia (mild bone loss) or osteoporosis

- Shakiness between meals

- Sleep disturbances

- Sugar cravings

- Thinning skin

- Weakened muscles

- Weakened immune system

- Weight gain

INSULIN

Insulin is a hormone produced by the pancreas. Its primary function is to regulate level of sugar (glucose) in your blood, though it is also believed to help repair damage to the body and stimulate muscle development.

Function in Memory and Cognition

Insulin plays several important roles in your brain, all of which can have a direct impact memory loss. Insulin receptors can be found throughout the brain, including in regions related to memory and cognition; their presence suggests that insulin can thus influence the proper functioning of these areas. Like estrogen, insulin is thought to help maintain your nerve synapses and regulate the growth, survival, and adaptation of existing brain cells. It also helps boost your brain's metabolism by supplying your neurons with the energy they need to function properly.

Because insulin is thus integral to proper brain function, abnormal levels of this important hormone can lead to memory loss and cognitive decline. Insulin levels can decline as a natural consequence of aging. They can also increase as part of a condition called insulin resistance, in which the body makes insulin but cannot process it, leading to high levels of unused insulin the bloodstream. Studies consistently show that both insulin deficiency and insulin resistance—a condition in which the body makes but cannot properly use insulin—can contribute to cognitive impairment and the degeneration of your brain's nerve cells, especially as these conditions relate to the development of Alzheimer's disease. People in the early stages of Alzheimer's disease often are seen to have lower levels of insulin in the brain and spinal fluid; as the symptoms of Alzheimer's disease progress, so, too, do insulin levels continue to drop. People with diabetes, a condition that is characterized by insulin resistance, have been shown to be 100 percent to 150 percent more likely to develop any type of dementia, and 50 percent to 100 percent more likely to develop Alzheimer's disease. Research also shows that even in people who do not have diabetes, elevated blood sugar levels (a symptom of insulin resistance) and diminished glycemic control are associated with cognitive decline.

While scientists are not sure of the exact mechanism that drives the relationship between insulin resistance and Alzheimer's disease, they suspect that it has to do with the connection between insulin and amyloid-B protein, a substance that in low amounts can enhance memory but in high amounts can contribute to the development of Alzheimer's disease. Researchers have observed that both insulin and amyloid-B protein are degraded by the same enzyme. At elevated levels (as in insulin resistance), insulin is processed and removed by this insulin-degrading enzyme (IDE), thus leaving less of the enzyme to break down amyloid-B protein. As a result, amyloid-B proteins build up to pathological levels that may cause memory decline, oxidative damage, and the formation of insoluble plaques. In other words, high insulin levels inhibit the degradation of amyloid-B protein, thus potentially contributing to the development of Alzheimer's disease.

As with all hormones, insulin must be kept at optimal levels—not too high and not too low—in order to prevent cognitive dysfunction. Low levels of insulin are also linked to memory loss. Studies have shown that in Alzheimer's patients who demonstrate low levels of insulin, both short-term and long-term insulin therapy improved memory and cognitive function. While more research must be done to determine whether insulin therapy confers benefits to people who suffer memory loss as a result of diabetes, high blood glucose levels, or aging, early results are promising.

Symptoms of Insulin Deficiency

- Bone loss
- Depression

- Fatigue
- Insomnia

Symptoms of Excess Insulin/Insulin Resistance

- Acne
- Aging process accelerates
- Asthma
- Breast cancer
- Colon cancer
- Depression and mood swings
- Estrogen levels that are too low
- Heart disease
- Heartburn

- High blood pressure
- High cholesterol
- High triglycerides
- Infertility
- Insomnia
- Irritable bowel syndrome
- Migraine headaches
- Osteopenia/osteoporosis
- Weight gain

MELATONIN

Melatonin is a hormone that is primarily produced by the pineal gland. Its main function is to help regulate your circadian rhythms—in particular, your twenty-four hour sleep-wake cycle. Recent studies suggest that melatonin may also be involved in your body's mechanisms of consciousness, memory, and stress. Animal studies indicate that melatonin may help protect your brain cells from the toxic effects of the heavy metal cobalt and amyloid B-protein, two substances that contribute to the development of Alzheimer's disease. In addition, low melatonin levels are linked to chronic sleep disorders and insomnia—issues that can contribute heavily to memory loss, as you will read in Chapter 6. While patients with Alzheimer's disease consistently show lower levels of this important hormone, more research needs to be done to determine whether melatonin replacement would be an advantageous treatment for Alzheimer's disease and other forms of cognitive decline.

Symptoms of Melatonin Deficiency

- Insomnia

- Compromised immune system

THYROID HORMONES

The thyroid gland produces two important hormones—triiodothyronine (T3) and thyroxine (T4)—both of which are primarily engaged in regulating metabolism and growth. Your body makes almost twenty times as much T4 as it does T3, though T3 is considered to be five times more potent (active) than T4. As a result, most of T4 is converted into T3 in your liver and kidneys. When your body takes in too much T4 through diet or supplements, T4 can also be converted into reverse T3, which is an inactive (stored) form.

Production of both T3 and T4 is regulated by thyroid-stimulating hormone (TSH), which is made in your pituitary gland. Like most hormones, T3, T4, and TSH all decline with age, though abnormal levels can also result from a variety of causes, including autoimmune disorders, thyroid surgeries, medications, and improper thyroid hormone replacement therapy.

Function in Memory and Cognition

Scientists have observed that hypothyroidism (low thyroid function) can lead to impaired nerve cell generation in the hippocampus (the brain's memory center), behavioral alterations, and cognitive deficits. Thyroid hormones may serve to support long-term potentiation (LTP), a process by which memories are formed; animal studies suggest that low levels of thyroid hormones are associated with impairment of LTP, and thus of memory. In addition, evidence suggests that thyroid hormones influence the maturation of the cholinergic system, which helps govern the learning process. Separately, low levels of thyroid-stimulating hormone (TSH) are believed to indicate risk of vascular dementia.

Although more research needs to be done on the benefits of thyroid hormone replacement therapy for memory and cognition, preliminary studies indicate that T4 replacement therapy can enhance learning ability and recall.

Some Symptoms of Thyroid Hormone Deficiency

- Cold hands and feet
- Constipation
- Decreased sexual interest

- Depression
- Fatigue
- Fluid retention

- High cholesterol

- High insulin levels

- Hoarse, husky voice

- Hypoglycemia (low blood sugar)

- Increased appetite

- Insomnia

- Intolerance to cold temperatures

- Loss of hair (varying amounts) from legs, armpit, and arms

- Menstrual irregularities

- Muscle cramps, pain, or weakness

- Poor circulation

- Reduced heart rate

- Rough, dry skin

- Swollen body, especially the legs, feet, hands, and abdomen

- Weight gain

VITAMIN D

Vitamin D is not really a vitamin at all, but rather a prohormone—a parent or "precursor" substance from which hormones can be synthesized. Several dietary sources are rich in vitamin D, including fish and fish liver oil, sweet potatoes, and dairy products, but it can also be made by your body when your skin is exposed to sunlight. The main functions of vitamin D are to help your body absorb calcium and mineralize (harden) bone. Vitamin D receptors are found throughout your body—in your bones, intestines, and, perhaps most notably, in your brain.

Vitamin D seems to play a role in regulating nerve transmissions, stimulating nerve cell generation. Studies suggest that vitamin D may thus help protect against neurodegenerative disorders, including Alzheimer's disease. While more research needs to be done, some initial studies have indicated that low vitamin D levels might be associated with cognitive impairment and a decline in spatial memory. Other studies have shown that increased vitamin D intake helped improve cognitive performance and skills.

Symptoms of Vitamin D Deficiency

- Fatigue

- Muscle or bone pain

PARATHYROID HORMONE

Parathyroid hormone (PTH) is produced by the four parathyroid glands in your neck. Although the main function of parathyroid hormone is to control blood levels of calcium, overproduction of parathyroid hormone (hyperparathyroidism) is frequently associated with dementia. In patients who suffer hyperparathyroidism, parathyroid therapy may improve or arrest memory loss.

Symptoms of Excess Parathyroid Hormone

- Abdominal pain

- Bone and joint pain

- Depression

- Excessive urination

- Fatigue or exhaustion

- Kidney stones

- Nausea or vomiting

- Osteoporosis or fragile bones

LEPTIN

Leptin is a hormone made by the body's fat cells. Its primary function is to regulate appetite and energy intake, but scientists increasingly believe it may also play a role in learning, memory, and brain development. While the greatest number of leptin receptors are found in the hypothalamus, the part of your brain that controls your metabolism, there are also high numbers of leptin receptors in the neocortex and the hippocampus, two areas of the brain that are responsible for the consolidation and maintenance of long-term memory. This suggests that leptin contributes to this memory-forming process—an idea that is supported by studies showing that Alzheimer's patients frequently demonstrate lower levels of leptin when compared with a control group. Other studies have shown the inverse to also be true: that older patients with higher leptin levels consistently exhibit less cognitive decline than patients with lower levels. More research needs to be done to determine whether leptin replacement would be an advantageous treatment for cognitive decline.

Symptoms of Leptin Deficiency

Because there is relatively little research on leptin, medical science has not yet established the definitive symptoms associated with leptin deficiency; weight gain is perhaps the symptom most commonly known.

DIAGNOSING HORMONAL IMBALANCES

Based on what you have just read, if you suspect that you have a hormonal imbalance, or that you are at risk for developing one, it is time to take action. First, consult with your doctor for further instruction. Most likely, you will then be advised to undergo hormone testing in order to give your doctor a better sense of which hormones you lack and which you have in excess. Only by determining the specific levels of your hormones can your doctor create a hormone replacement therapy that is right for your needs.

Hormone levels should be evaluated before beginning hormone replacement therapy, and then re-evaluated three months after. Thereafter, hormone levels should be tested routinely, or as your doctor prescribes.

In this section, we describe the three most common methods used to test hormone levels and imbalances.

Saliva Tests

Saliva, or salivary, testing, is the method of hormone testing most frequently recommended by healthcare providers. Available for all three forms of estrogen, progesterone, testosterone, cortisol, and DHEA, salivary testing measures the level of "free" hormones in your saliva—that is, the precise amount of each hormone that is considered active and available for immediate use. In contrast to serum (blood) testing, salivary testing reflects the hormone levels throughout the entire body. Easily ordered online, saliva tests are convenient and noninvasive; you complete the tests in the privacy of your home, and then send the samples back to the lab for quick and accurate results.

Urine Tests

Another excellent method for evaluating hormonal function is the twenty-four-hour urine test. Like salivary testing, urinary testing offers a simple, noninvasive way to evaluate your free hormone levels over time. The procedure for urine testing is simple. You will be asked to collect all your urine in a specially provided container over a twenty-four hour period. After twenty-four hours have elapsed, you will then send the urine to a lab for analysis.

One advantage to this form of testing is that in addition to testing free hormone levels, urine tests also measure the amounts of metabolites, or breakdown products, of various sex hormones. This allows your doctor to obtain a more complete picture of how your hormones are produced and used—not only by your endocrine system, but also by peripheral organs and glands.

Blood Tests

Unlike saliva and urine tests, blood tests measure the total volume of both free and "bound" (stored or unavailable) levels of certain hormones in your bloodstream. Because some blood tests do not differentiate between free and bound forms, and because they only test these levels at a single point in time, however, their efficacy in measuring cortisol and sex hormones is limited. Blood tests are often used to test thyroid hormones, pregnenolone, and insulin. Most blood tests require only a single blood draw, from which the lab can perform all its analyses.

TREATMENT OPTIONS FOR HORMONAL IMBALANCES

Scientific technology has developed to a point where it is now viable to rectify hormonal imbalances. If hormone testing reveals a deficiency or excess, your doctor may recommend that you consider hormone replacement therapy (HRT). By optimizing your hormone levels, you will be better equipped to ward off memory loss and cognitive decline.

Until a few decades ago, the only hormonal therapy available in the United States was synthetic hormone replacement.

Synthetic Hormone Replacement Therapy

Synthetic hormones are laboratory-produced hormones that mimic the effects of hormones that exist naturally within your body. Although the effects may be similar, however, a synthetic hormone has a very different chemical structure from a natural or bioidentical hormone—this is what makes it "synthetic."

Because synthetic hormones aren't equivalent to the ones your body produces, their benefits are limited. In fact, evidence increasingly shows that synthetic hormones can actually be harmful. In 2002, the government-sponsored Women's Health Initiative Program published a study indicating that synthetic hormones increased risk of heart disease, osteoporosis, and certain types of cancer in women who had not had a hysterectomy. Follow-up studies largely confirmed the findings of the Women's Health Initiative, noting in addition that one-half of all women undergoing synthetic hormone replacement therapy dropped out after a year due to the unpleasant side effects.

Fortunately, there is an alternative to synthetic hormone replacement therapy.

Natural (Bioidentical) Hormone Replacement Therapy

Like synthetic hormones, many natural hormones are actually made in the laboratory. The difference between the two types of hormones comes from the fact that natural hormones are *bioidentical*—that is, their chemical structures are exactly the same as the ones made by your body. As a result, these bioidentical hormones are more readily accepted for use by your brain and other organs, making them the hormones of choice for most doctors.

But it is not enough to simply take bioidentical hormones instead of synthetic ones. One size does not fit all. In the past, doctors have assumed that a standardized dosage was appropriate for rectifying any hormonal imbalance. This approach may do more harm than good. Instead, use the Resources section to find a doctor who will customize your natural hormone replacement therapy to your precise needs, using compounded—individually calibrated—hormones that are derived from plant extracts. Your hormone response is as unique to you as your fingerprints are. Each person's hormone requirements are different, and depend on a variety of factors, including genetic profile, stress level, health condition, environment, nutritional supplementation, and diet. Only by tailoring your hormone therapy to your specific needs can you achieve the results you require to remedy and prevent memory loss.

CONCLUSION

Having read this chapter, you now have a better understanding of how important hormones are to the proper functioning of your brain, and what can happen when these hormones get out of balance. Because hormones are integral to maintaining and supporting your cognitive ability, an excess or deficiency of these essential chemicals can have serious consequences for your mental acuity. Memory loss can often be a sign of hormonal imbalance. Fortunately, it is now possible to rectify these imbalances–and any related memory loss—through judicious use of natural hormone replacement therapy. Consult with your doctor in order to get started on a regimen that can have enormous benefits for your mind!

Is Your Memory Loss Caused by Inflammation?

This test was designed to help you determine whether inflammation might be affecting your memory and cognition. Read each question carefully and place a check mark in the box that best represents your answer.

	Yes	No	Unsure
1. Do you suffer from gas, bloating, or indigestion?	☐	☐	☐
2. Do you have food allergies or intolerances?	☐	☐	☐
3. Do you suffer from a gastrointestinal disorder such as inflammatory bowel disorder or leaky gut syndrome?	☐	☐	☐
4. Do you eat a diet that is high in sugars and processed food?	☐	☐	☐
5. Are you overweight by twenty pounds or more?	☐	☐	☐
6. Are you prone to infections?	☐	☐	☐
7. Do you use antacids on a regular basis?	☐	☐	☐
8. Do you smoke?	☐	☐	☐
9. Do you take oral estrogen supplements?	☐	☐	☐
10. Are you exposed to heavy metals (aluminum, mercury, lead) on a regular basis?	☐	☐	☐

If you answered "yes" to any of these questions, your memory loss may be the result of chronic inflammation!

5

Inflammation

Chronic or long-term inflammation is the culprit in many cases of memory impairment. Inflammation is essentially an immune response, your body's way of defending itself against harm—bacterial infections, damage from toxins, or physical trauma. When appropriate, inflammation is a process that allows your body to heal itself. But over the long term, inflammation can damage your brain cells, making it difficult for them to function properly and leading to impaired memory and cognition.

To understand how this happens, let's take a closer look at the inflammatory process. There are two types of inflammation: acute and chronic. Acute, or short-term, inflammation occurs as a reaction to an immediate injury or threat. Within seconds of cutting your finger, for example, your body releases certain chemicals, including histamine, bradykinin, cytokines, and prostaglandins. These chemicals mediate, or regulate, the inflammatory response, widening your blood vessels and rushing blood cells, proteins, and other healing compounds to the affected area to repair the damage. In particular, white blood cells—your body's natural defenders—rally to attack invaders (bacteria or toxins), and to either neutralize or "eat" dead and damaged cells, eradicating the threat. Because of the increased blood flow, the region around the cut swells and turns red, and you feel heat and pain as the swollen tissue exerts pressure on your nerves. This minor discomfort is a good sign: it means that the damage is being quarantined and restored, allowing for new, healthy tissue to take its place.

Acute inflammation is a beneficial and tightly orchestrated event that continues only as long as it takes to protect your body from further harm and initiate the repair process. By contrast, chronic (long-term) inflammation occurs when an acute inflammation response fails to heal or resolve an injury, or in response to progressive damage or prolonged exposure to a toxic substance. Sometimes chronic inflammation can occur even when no harmful or invasive agent is present. During chronic inflammation, your body keeps trying to defend itself against a perceived threat—regardless of whether one exists—and ends up attacking and destroying its own tissue, both damaged and healthy.

The results can be devastating for your brain. In essence, inflammation anywhere in the body can indirectly cause inflammation in the brain. This is because the cytokines and other substances that cause localized inflammations (in the gastrointestinal tract, for example) can travel through the blood stream to the central nervous system, where they stimulate the production of new cytokines that travel to the brain. There, they initiate new inflammation, causing damage to your neurons that can lead to memory loss, cognitive decline, and even psychological problems like depression.

The questionnaire at the beginning of the chapter is designed to help you determine whether chronic inflammation is affecting your memory and focus. If you answered "yes" to any of the questions, you may be suffering from chronic inflammation, and thus inflammation-related cognitive impairment. This chapter will educate you as to the symptoms, causes, and risk factors of chronic inflammation, so that you will be better able to treat or prevent this debilitating condition. In turn, by reducing or warding off inflammation, you may potentially be reducing or warding off cognitive decline.

To learn how to recognize chronic inflammation, you must first be able to identify the most common symptoms associated with this condition.

SYMPTOMS

Because it often affects internal organs, chronic inflammation usually lacks the obvious symptoms that characterize acute inflammation (redness, swelling). Moreover, symptoms of chronic inflammation can be nonspecific—meaning that they occur in a variety of disorders or conditions—and can vary according to the area of the body affected.

Besides memory impairment or cognitive decline, there are many other symptoms that may signal chronic inflammation. Below, you will find a list of general symptoms, followed by more specific categories of symptoms that may occur, depending on the type of inflammatory disorder experienced and the area of the body affected.

General Symptoms of Chronic Inflammation

- Body aches and pains
- Chronic diarrhea
- Nasal congestion
- Shortness of breath
- Chronic indigestion
- Skin outbreaks

- Dry eyes
- Stiffness of joints
- Fluid retention
- Swelling of joints
- Frequent infection
- Weight gain/obesity

Allergic or Respiratory Symptoms

- Asthma
- Bronchitis (recurrent)
- Burning or tingling of the extremities
- Chemical sensitivity
- Coughing
- Fatigue
- Hay fever
- Headache

- Itchy skin, eyes, or nose
- Muscle or joint pain or weakness
- Nasal congestion
- Nausea
- Shortness of breath
- Sinusitis (sinus infection)
- Sore throat
- Tremors

Cognitive and Emotional Symptoms

- Anxiety
- Confusion
- Delirium
- Delusions
- Depression
- Disorientation

- Hyperactivity
- Inability to concentrate
- Irritability
- Mood swings
- Nervousness
- Obsessive-compulsive behavior

Gastrointestinal Symptoms

- Bloating

- Cramps

- Diarrhea

- Dyspepsia

- Food sensitivities

- Gas

- Heartburn

- Increased reflux

- Lactose intolerance

- Vitamin deficiencies

  - Fat soluble vitamins (A,D, E, K)

  - Iron

  - Vitamins B_9 and B_{12}

  - Calcium

- Weight loss

- Weight gain

CAUSES AND RISK FACTORS

Currently a hot topic among medical researchers, inflammation is considered an underlying factor in a host of serious health problems, including rheumatoid arthritis, lupus, heart disease, obesity, type 2 diabetes, and even cancer. In turn, chronic inflammation itself can be caused by a number of conditions and disorders. Below, you will find several of the primary causes and risk factors of chronic inflammation. While it can often be difficult to isolate the precise source of inflammation—particularly since scientists are still struggling to understand the full significance of this problem—by identifying some of the better-known causes, this chapter will prepare you to take action to treat or prevent them.

Food Allergies and Intolerances

Food intolerances can be a major source of chronic inflammation, particularly if they go unrecognized for long periods of time. Over 60 percent of all Americans suffer from some sort of food reaction, varying in severity from a food sensitivity (mild symptoms), intolerance (moderate symptoms), or allergy (serious symptoms). Because there is often some confusion amongst the public about the difference between allergies and intolerances, it is useful to explain what these two reactions are.

A food allergy will cause your immune system to react immediately and severely in response to even the smallest particle of the offending substance: your mouth may tingle or swell, or you might break out in hives, vomit, or feel nauseated. In extreme cases, you may go into ana-phylaxis—a sometimes fatal condition characterized by very low blood pressure and the inability to breathe.

By contrast, food intolerance is less likely to be life-threatening, developing more gradually over time, often as the result of a lack of appropriate digestive enzymes. Food intolerance is considered an auto-immune disorder. That is, whereas in a food allergy, your immune sys-tem attacks a nutrient that it would ordinarily ignore, in food intolerance, when you eat a problematic food, your immune system attacks your body itself.

For people who suffer from gluten intolerance or its more severe rela-tion, celiac disease, consumption of gluten (a protein found in wheat, rye, and barley) causes the immune system to destroy parts of the small intes-tine and gastrointestinal (GI) tract. This destruction sets off an inflamma-tory response as your immune system tries to heal the damage; unless gluten is quickly removed from the diet, this inflammation can become chronic.

While digestive problems—including diarrhea, cramps, bloating, and indigestion—are usually the first signs of this gastrointestinal inflamma-tion, a decline in cognition is not uncommon. Scientists don't yet under-stand what causes gluten intolerance and celiac disease to create neurological and psychiatric problems, but some suspect that the blame lies with nutritional deficiencies caused by the damaged GI tract's dimin-ished ability to absorb nutrients. Deprived of the nutrients they need to work properly, brain cells begin to malfunction and die, leading to mem-ory loss and other cognitive problems.

Gastrointestinal Disorders

Gluten intolerance and celiac disease are not the only gastrointestinal dis-orders to affect the brain. Because the brain depends on the digestive sys-tem to absorb and process the energy and nutrients it needs in order to function, any condition that compromises the gastrointestinal tract thus also potentially endangers your cognitive ability.

One of the most common gastrointestinal sources of inflammation is dysbiosis, or an imbalance of bacteria in the digestive tract. Your gut is home to over 1,000 different species of bacteria. When these bacteria are maintained in proper amounts within your intestinal lining, they perform many useful tasks, helping to protect the gut, digest your food, and support your immune function. But when the bacteria get out of balance as the result of poor nutrition, long-term use of antacids and other medications, excessive alcohol intake, low levels of digestive enzymes or stomach acid, viruses, or other injurious agents, your GI tract becomes vulnerable to damage and infection. And once the GI tract is damaged, your body quickly sets off an inflammatory response to heal the damage.

The trouble is, it's often difficult to resolve dysbiosis, and so inflammation can become a chronic or sustained issue. Dysbiosis has been linked to the development of three other debilitating GI disorders: leaky gut syndrome, inflammatory bowel disease (IBD), and ulcerative colitis. If you suffer from any of these problems, you essentially have a chronic inflammatory condition, as all three are characterized by significant inflammation of the GI tract. Leaky gut syndrome can be particularly worrisome for cognition, as the inflammation involved actually makes the intestines more permeable, not less, allowing toxins and other damaging substances to travel through the bloodstream and causing systemic inflammation. That is to say, the inflammation involved in GI disorders is not localized; it can spread to all areas of your body, including your brain—where it can inflict serious damage.

Heavy Metals And Other Toxins

As discussed in Chapter 3, heavy metals and other toxins can directly hurt your ability to think and recall information. They can also indirectly impact cognition by contributing to chronic inflammation, as any foreign substance that is introduced to your body can potentially set off a critical immune response. Particularly notorious offenders include heavy metals such as aluminum, arsenic, lead, and mercury. Because these metals are extremely toxic, causing damage to your heart, kidneys, immune system, bones, and nerves, your body treats them as invaders, initiating an inflammatory response that can turn chronic if these substances are not quickly eradicated from your system.

Infections

When you are infected by a bacteria, virus, fungus, or parasite, your body initiates an inflammatory response to fight off the intruder. Unfortunately, sometimes infections can be hard to eradicate; in these cases, chronic inflammation develops as your body persistently tries to get rid of the enemy. Examples of inflammation-causing infections include:

- *Parasitic infections.* Microscopic parasites can take up residence in the intestinal walls, where they breed and develop into widespread infestations, causing inflammation and disrupting normal digestive processes. Common parasite conditions include giardia, *Entamoeba histolytica*, cyclospora, or cryptosporidium infections.

- *Yeast infections.* The yeasts of the genus *Candida* are among billions of microorganisms found in the body's mucous membranes—in the mouth, throat, digestive tract, and genitals. Ordinarily, growth of these yeasts (which are actually fungi) is controlled by various factors within the body, but certain factors—including alcohol intake, use of certain medications, exposure to chemicals and toxins, pregnancy, and chronic stress—can cause them to increase beyond healthy levels. While they are commonly associated with vaginal infections, yeast infections can develop in both men and women and in many areas of the body (mouth, urinary tract, stomach). Moreover, yeast infections don't always limit themselves to a single location; they can spread through the bloodstream, producing systemic infections that affect the blood, esophagus, eyes, heart, kidneys, liver, skin, and spleen. They can even take up residence in the gastrointestinal tract, where they can contribute to the development of leaky gut syndrome and other digestive disorders. Wherever they go, the response is the same: inflammation develops in order to curb this rampant yeast overgrowth.

- *Lyme disease.* Lyme disease is a infection of the bacteria *Borrelia burgdorferi* (*B. burgdorferi*), which is commonly carried and spread by ticks and other insects. Left untreated, the bacteria can multiply and travel through the bloodstream to locations outside the original area of infection, potentially invading and damaging tendons, muscles, the heart, and the brain. In response to this damage, inflammation develops, often turning chronic as the infection can be difficult to eliminate if not treated immediately.

Oxidative Stress

Oxidative stress is a type of physiological stress that is caused by unstable oxygen compounds called free radicals. Ordinarily, special molecules called antioxidants help contain and neutralize free radicals, keeping them at appropriate levels. In small volumes, free radicals even perform some useful functions, helping with hormone synthesis, energy production, and signal transmission in neurons. But when the number of free radicals in your system increases—due to aging, stress, radiation, and exposure to toxins (alcohol, caffeine, sugar, cigarette smoke, heavy metals, pesticides, and other environmental pollutants)—these molecules turn dangerous, attacking and destroying cells and tissue throughout the body. As a result, inflammation sets in to heal the damage.

Independent of its inflammatory effects, oxidative stress has been linked to the development of many serious diseases due to its tendency to disrupt signal transmission between cells. In particular, oxidative stress is implicated in many neurodegenerative disorders, including Parkinson's disease, Alzheimer's disease, Lou Gehrig's disease (ALS), and Huntington's disease.

Weight Gain or Obesity

Strange as it may sound, being overweight or obese can contribute to chronic inflammation. Contrary to popular belief, adipose tissue (fat cells) doesn't just sit there, making you look chubby; it actually performs a number of tasks. Among other things, adipose tissue releases cytokines, which are special molecules that can initiate inflammation. The more cytokines that are released, the more intense (and chronic) the inflammation.

In turn, this inflammation can prevent your brain from responding to hormones that help regulate your metabolism and weight, including leptin, insulin, and cortisol (see Chapter 4). Accordingly, you put on pounds and develop even more adipose tissue, further escalating the production of cytokines. The result is a vicious circle of weight gain and inflammation that can be difficult to escape.

Other Causes and Risk Factors of Chronic Inflammation

As you can see, there are many causes and risk factors of inflammation, and more are being discovered every day. In addition to the problems discussed above, various other factors may play a role in either initiating or developing inflammation. They include:

- **Fatty Acid Imbalance.** A deficiency of omega-3 fatty acids (commonly found in fish oil) or an excess of omega-6 fatty acids (commonly found in palm, soy, and canola oil) can increase inflammation.

- **Oral Estrogen Therapy.** Oral estrogen therapy can increase inflammation and blood clotting; for this reason, estrogen should always be used transdermally (through the skin).

- **Physical Trauma (Cuts, Bruises, Broken Bones, etc.).** Chronic inflammation can develop out of an acute inflammatory response to an injury.

- **Smoking.** Cigarettes and other tobacco products can damage your lungs and other organs, leading to inflammation.

- **Sugar intake.** Consuming large amounts of refined sugar intake can trigger the release of cytokines and increase your levels of the inflammatory markers C-reactive protein (CRP) and interleukin 6 (IL-6).

- **Surgery.** Anything that injures or disrupts your cells and tissues—be it a simple tooth extraction or open-heart surgery—will initiate an inflammatory response, as your body attempts to heal the wound.

It's important to note that the different causes of inflammation can sometimes be interconnected. For example, heavy metal exposure is both a source of inflammation in its own right and as an instigator of oxidative stress; consumption of sugar and other harmful substances can stimulate inflammation and also contribute to weight gain, a separate source of inflammation. Clearly, inflammation is a complicated process, the full significance of which will only be revealed in time.

DIAGNOSIS

As we discussed earlier, chronic inflammation rarely announces itself with obvious symptoms. If you believe you might be suffering from chronic inflammation, it is time to visit a doctor. Because the causes of inflammation are so varied, your doctor is likely to prescribe a battery of tests that evaluate for the presence of different markers and thus allow you to pinpoint the source of your problems.

First, there are four general tests that your doctor may order to establish whether inflammation is present.

- **C-reactive Protein (CRP) Test**. This simple, common blood test measures your body's levels of C-reactive protein (CRP), a primary marker of inflammation throughout the body. High levels of this substance indicate a heightened state of inflammation—although low levels of C-reactive protein do not rule out the presence of inflammation. In addition to evaluating for the general presence of inflammation, special CRP tests are often used to evaluate the risk of coronary artery disease, which doctors now believe to be driven by inflammatory processes.

- **Erythrocyte Sedimentation Rate (ESR, or Sed Rate)**. This test measures the rate at which erythrocytes (red blood cells) sediment, or fall to the bottom of a test tube. Higher rates indicate the presence of inflammation, as certain proteins associated with inflammation will cause the red blood cells to stick together and sink faster.

- **Fasting Blood Insulin Test**. Typically used to screen for diabetes and heart disease, the fasting blood insulin test measures your body's levels of insulin, a hormone that allows your body to process glucose (sugar) for energy. Insulin can be a marker for inflammation. Accordingly, higher levels of insulin indicate the presence of systemic inflammation.

- **Inflammatory Cytokine Profile Test**. The most comprehensive of the tests, an inflammatory cytokine profile measures your body's levels of cytokines, the protein molecules that mediate (regulate) the inflammatory process. Cytokines evaluated include interleukins, interferons, and tumor necrosis factor; higher levels of any of these cytokines can indicate systemic inflammation.

If any of the above tests indicate the presence of inflammation, your doctor may then order more specialized tests to identify the source of the problem. The following are tests that can be used to confirm the specific cause of your inflammation.

Tests for Food Allergies or Intolerances

Currently, there are no scientific tests that can reliably establish the existence of a food intolerance. The best way to determine whether you have a sensitivity or intolerance to a substance is to simply eliminate it from your diet and see if inflammatory symptoms disappear.

While there is no standard test to confirm a food allergy, a variety of methods are available. The most common is the skin prick test. In it, small areas of your skin are scratched and then exposed to various allergens. The areas are then observed for swelling or other evidence of a reaction. A positive reaction, however, is not necessarily sufficient evidence of an allergy; for confirmation, other methods should also be used. Your doctor may also order an immunoglobin E (IgE) or immunoglobin G (IgG) test to evaluate for the presence of antibodies that specifically respond to allergens; unfortunately, neither test is reliable as a single indicator of an allergy.

As with food intolerance, the best way to test for a food allergy is probably the elimination method. Only by removing a substance completely from your diet can you determine whether it is the source of your inflammation and other health woes. Occasionally, these problem foods can even be reintroduced back into your diet after a sufficient period of time has elapsed.

Tests for Gastrointestinal Disorders

Because their exact causes still elude scientists, it can be difficult to definitively diagnose gastrointestinal disorders that are characterized by dysbiosis and inflammation, such as inflammatory bowel disease, ulcerative colitis, or leaky gut syndrome. Often, a diagnosis will be reached only by ruling out the presence of other (noninflammatory) gastrointestinal disorders, such as ischemic colitis, irritable bowel syndrome (IBS), diverticulitis, or colon cancer.

Tests that can be used to help confirm a diagnosis of inflammatory bowel disease or ulcerative colitis include:

- **Blood Test**. Primarily used to determine the presence of anemia or infection, blood tests can also be employed to scan for certain antibodies that are implicated in specific types of GI inflammation.

- **Colonoscopy**. In this test, a thin flexible tube with a tiny camera attached to it is threaded through the colon (large intestine), allowing your doctor to see any polyps, damage, or inflammation that might be present. Tissue samples can also be taken for laboratory analysis.

- **Computed Tomography (CT) Scan**. Using x-rays, a CT scan provides a complete picture of your abdomen, and can indicate the presence and intensity of inflammation there.

- **Flexible Sigmoidscopy**. In this test, a thin, flexible tube is used to examine the sigmoid colon, which is the part of the colon closest to the rectum and anus. Because it does not examine the entire colon, flexible sigmoidscopy is used only when inflammation is too extensive to safely and comfortably perform a colonoscopy.

- **Stool Sample**. A stool sample is analyzed to evaluate for the presence of white blood cells, which can indicate inflammation, or for bacterial imbalances that indicate dysbiosis. Specialized testing can also look for problems with digestion, such as a lack of digestive enzymes. Stool samples can also be used to rule out parasites or yeast as a potential cause of symptoms.

Tests for Exposure to Heavy Metals and Other Toxins

Since the symptoms of heavy metal poisoning and other forms of toxic buildup are nonspecific (that is, similar to the symptoms of other dis--orders and conditions), it can be difficult to know that you are suffering from these conditions and thus take the appropriate measures. When appropriate, blood and urine tests can be performed to evaluate your levels of these toxic substances. For more information, see Chapter 3.

Tests for Infections

Generally, an infection can be diagnosed if a blood test indicates high levels of white blood cells, your body's first defense against bacteria and other infectious agents. Tests to confirm the specific source of an infection vary according to the suspected culprit.

Parasitic infections are commonly diagnosed with a stool sample, which is analyzed for the presence of different microorganisms. Yeast infections can sometimes be diagnosed by visual clues alone, but confirmation of *Candida* overgrowth can be received through the analysis of stool samples or a blood test called the Candida Immune Complex Assay, which evaluates for the presence of certain antibodies that specifically fight yeast. Lyme disease is typically diagnosed with the enzyme-linked immunosorbent assay (ELISA) test, a blood test that scans for the presence of antibodies that whose purpose is to fight *B. burgdorferi*, the bacteria that causes the disease. A new test called the iSpot Lyme test is also available (see Resources).

Tests for Oxidative Stress

Because oxidative stress is still a topic of much debate among researchers, there is no definitive clinical test to measure it. Often, laboratories will instead measure the levels of antioxidants in the body; low levels indicate that supplies of these important substances have been depleted in the attempt to combat a greater number of free radicals, the cause of oxidative stress. Antioxidants measured include glutathione (GSH), glutathione peroxidase (GPx), and superoxide dismutase (SOD).

Tests for Obesity

The best way to evaluate whether you are overweight or obese is to determine your body mass index (BMI). The BMI is a measure of body fat based on height and weight. To calculate your BMI, divide your weight in pounds by your height in inches, squared, then multiply this number by 703:

$$\frac{\text{Your Weight}}{\text{Your Height times Your Height}} \times 703 = \text{Your Body Mass Index}$$

If the resulting number is between 18.5 and 25, you are of normal weight. A BMI between 25 is considered overweight, and anything above 30 is classified as obese.

TREATMENT

Fortunately, it possible to prevent, reduce, and even eradicate inflammation. The important thing is to eliminate all the external sources of inflammation, or as many as you can. If you are suffering from an infection, heavy metal poisoning, or a gastrointestinal disorder, talk with your doctor to create a strategy that will help clear up these conditions.

More generally, get rid of those toxins! Limit your exposure to heavy metals and fluoride, quit smoking, and avoid radiation and surgery if at all possible.

Restore Your Digestive Health

Next, eliminate any food-based toxins from your diet. If you suspect you have a food allergy or intolerance, or if you suffer from a digestive condition brought on by dysbiosis, immediate action should be taken to restore the health of your gastrointestinal tract. Follow the "Four R Program" developed by Dr. Jeffrey Bland of the Functional Medicine Institute:

- **Remove** the source of any allergy, intolerance, or imbalance. To be safe, you may want to eliminate all common allergy-producing foods from your diet, particularly gluten and dairy products. Abstain entirely from substances that can irritate or damage the lining of your intestines, including alcohol, caffeine, and nonsteroidal anti-inflammatory drugs (aspirin, ibuprofen, naproxen, etc.).

- **Replace** stomach acid and digestive enzymes depleted by aging, overuse of antacids, and heavy metal exposure. Low levels of stomach acid and digestive enzymes may contribute to dysbiosis and prevent you from processing and absorbing your food properly. Bitter substances, such as dandelion greens, escarole, endive, or extracts of ginger, cardamom, and fennel seed, can help replenish supplies of both acid and digestive enzymes.

- **Repopulate** your gut's bacteria colonies. As discussed earlier, a good balance of stomach bacteria is essential to ensure proper digestion. By taking probiotics—microbes that encourage normal levels of the right bacteria—you can soon restore your GI tract to optimal health. Probiotics like *Lactobacilli* and *Bifidobacteria* can be found in most yogurts, or taken separately as supplements. You can also consume prebiotics, which are substances that act as food for probiotics, helping fuel their growth. Prebiotics can be found in Jerusalem artichokes, onions, asparagus, and garlic; prebiotic supplements include fructooligosaccharides (FOS), arabinogalactans, active immunoglobulins from whey, lactoferrin, and lactoperoxidase.

- **Repair** any damage done to the GI tract by supplying it with nutrients that aid its recovery. In particular, try adding glutamine supplements to your diet. This important amino acid protects and stimulates the growth of the beneficial mucous lining that coats your intestines; it also helps create a favorable acid-alkaline balance in your stomach. You can also try quercetin, vitamin A, vitamin C, and vitamin E; all of these supplements act as antioxidants and anti-inflammatories.

Diet

Once you have restored the balance of your digestive system, you must work hard to maintain it. Because the standard American diet is probably the main contributor to most cases of chronic inflammation, any attempt to control inflammation should necessarily involve a change in eating habits. This is particularly true for people whose chronic inflammation stems from food intolerance or a gastrointestinal disorder. Besides identifying and or removing any problematic foods from your diet, many doctors now recommend following a Mediterranean-style diet for optimal nutrition and health. Studies have shown that even one day on the Mediterranean diet can lower levels of CRP, one of the primary markers of inflammation (see above). In addition, the Mediterranean diet supports cardiovascular health and weight loss. For a general overview of the Mediterranean diet, see Chapter 12.

Supplements

In addition to improving your diet, you can also supplement your intake of inflammation-fighting nutrients with supplements. The following table lists various supplements commonly used to reduce inflammation and promote overall health.

Supplement	Dosage	Considerations
Bromelain	250 mg twice a day.	Do not take if you are allergic to pineapple, from which this enzyme is derived.
Garlic (*Allium sativum*)	400 mg twice a day.	Do not take if you are on a blood-thinning medication.
Ginger root (*Zingiber officinale*)	500 mg twice a day.	Do not take if you are on a blood-thinning medication or NSAIDs. If you have allergies or problems with your heart, nervous system, or kidneys, consult with your healthcare professional before taking.
Ginkgo (*Ginkgo biloba*)	120 mg once a day.	Do not take if you are on a blood-thinning medication.
Glucosamine	500 to 1,000 mg three times a day.*	Do not take if you are allergic to shellfish. Consult with your healthcare provider if you have diabetes, because glucosamine can alter blood sugar levels.

*To choose an appropriate dose, see page 157 for information on dosage ranges.

Supplement	Dosage	Considerations
Grape seed extract and pycnogenol	50 mg twice a day.	Consult with your healthcare provider if you have diabetes or hypoglycemia (low blood sugar; take cholesterol-lowering medications; have a history of bleeding or clotting disorders; or take blood-thinning medications, NSAIDS, antiplatelet medications, blood pressure medications, or medications that stimulate or suppress the immune system.
Green tea or Green tea extract	1 cup three times a day (tea), or 250 mg one to two times a day (extract).	Green tea may increase the risk of bleeding if you are taking aspirin or other blood-thinning medications. If tea causes heartburn or acid reflux, drink it with a meal.
Methylsulfonyl-methane (MSM)	1,000 to 3,000 mg three times a day.*	Consult with your healthcare provider if you have kidney disease, liver disease, or an ulcer. High doses can deplete your body of B-complex vitamins.
Milk thistle (*Silybum marianum*)	100 to 200 mg twice a day	May reduce the effectiveness of birth control pills.
Omega-3 fatty acids EPA/DHA (fish oil)	2,000 to 10,000 mg once a day.*	Do not take more than 4,000 mg if you are also taking a blood-thinning medication; omega-3 fatty acids may increase effects.
Quercetin	200 to 500 mg once a day.*	If supplement causes heartburn or acid reflux, take it with a meal.
Trans-resveratrol	200 mg once a day.	To avoid additives such as caffeine, look for a product that is 99 percent trans-resveratrol.
Turmeric curcuminoids	300 mg twice a day.	May cause an upset stomach or heartburn; can also increase the risk of kidney stones.

*To choose an appropriate dose, see page 157 for information on dosage ranges.

Exercise

Exercise is a safe and inexpensive form of anti-inflammatory medicine. When you exercise, your body releases special substances that control inflammation and help repair and regenerate tissue. Some experts believe that the lack of physical activity in contemporary society is responsible for the increased rates of inflammatory disorders such as asthma, heart disease, diabetes, and cancer. It's important not to overexert yourself, though; excessive exercise can actually damage your body, causing an inflammatory response. The key is to exercise consistently and moderately; by maintaining a healthy level of physical fitness, you can decrease your risk of chronic inflammation. Moreover, as you will see in Chapter 8, exercise is independently beneficial for cognition and memory.

CONCLUSION

Chronic inflammation is a major issue in the United States, underlying many serious diseases and disorders. As you have seen, there are also many causes or risk factors that contribute to this debilitating condition. Although there is still much we don't know about the exact mechanisms that drive the inflammatory process, the effects of chronic inflammation on memory and cognition are clear and hazardous. Fortunately, there are lots of ways you can reduce or even prevent chronic inflammation from taking hold of your body—and thus your mind! By limiting or avoiding exposure to toxins, and by eating right and exercising, you can control your risk of inflammation and ensure that your mind will never suffer because of it.

Is Your Memory Loss Caused by Insomnia?

This test was designed to help you determine whether insomnia might be affecting your memory and cognition. Read each question carefully and place a check mark in the box that best represents your answer.

	Yes	No	Unsure
1. Do you regularly sleep fewer than seven hours each night?	☐	☐	☐
2. Does it usually take more than half an hour for you to fall asleep?	☐	☐	☐
3. Do you have trouble getting to sleep three nights or more each week?	☐	☐	☐
4. Have your sleep issues lasted for a month or longer?	☐	☐	☐
5. Do you wake up several times during the night?	☐	☐	☐
5a. If so, does it take you a long time to get back to sleep afterwards?	☐	☐	☐
6. Do you regularly wake up earlier in the morning than you'd prefer?	☐	☐	☐
7. When you wake up, do you still feel tired?	☐	☐	☐
8. Do you have trouble staying awake during the day?	☐	☐	☐
9. Has your fatigue begun to interfere with your work, family, or social life?	☐	☐	☐
10. Are you under a lot of stress?	☐	☐	☐

If you answered "yes" to the majority of these questions, your memory loss may be the result of chronic insomnia!

6

Insomnia

As anybody who has ever pulled an all-nighter can attest, lack of sleep can result in significant lapses in memory and focus. But what happens to your cognitive ability when you get little or light sleep for extended periods of time? In the United States today, it is estimated that over a quarter of the population has experienced some form of insomnia—a condition that is defined as difficulty in either falling asleep or staying asleep—with nearly ten percent of all Americans suffering from chronic (long-term) insomnia. This figure is troubling. While sleep deprivation can generally produce negative consequences for your entire body, poor or inadequate sleep can seriously impair your focus and memory.

This is because under normal circumstances, sleep aids memory consolidation, the process by which long-term memories are formed and stabilized. During the day, you accumulate new information and experiences, each of which leaves a neural trace—a new pathway between neurons—in your brain. Consolidation allows the new data and events to be fixed in your mind so that you can recall them at a later time. Although memories are constantly being consolidated as new information is taken in, research has shown that this process is most active and intensive during sleep. When you sleep, your brain also makes decisions about which memories to retain or discard. Recently, studies have suggested that different stages of sleep are associated with the stabilization of different types of memories.

Moreover, sleep not only helps you secure your memories, but also sets the stage for the formation of these memories in the first place, allowing for better acquisition of new knowledge during the day. Research indicates that if you haven't slept, your ability to learn declines by as much as 40 percent.

Because both sleep and memory are incredibly complex processes, scientists are still working to understand exactly how they interact. Sleep generally provides opportunities for your body to repair and recondition itself. Accordingly, many believe that sleep promotes the construction of new pathways between your brain cells, literally allowing for fresh connections and associations to be formed in your mind. At the same time, recent research suggests that the opposite also occurs: that when you sleep, certain connections between your neurons are selectively weakened or destroyed, allowing your brain to conserve energy by winnowing out your memories to just the most powerful or important.

In addition, sleep encourages the production of many hormones that help you maintain your memory, as discussed in Chapter 4. Among the hormones made during sleep is growth hormone, the hormone that keeps you young by restoring and regenerating your body's cells—including your brain cells. Sleep also helps reduce levels of free radicals, molecules associated with aging that can damage your brain cells and inhibit cognitive function.

Without sleep, your body is less capable of performing the protective and restorative processes that allow your brain to consolidate memories. Studies have consistently shown that chronic sleep deprivation increases the aging process in the brain and causes damage to the neurons, leading to serious memory decline.

Thus if you or a loved one suffer from impaired memory or focus, it could be the result of chronic insomnia or another sleep disorder. The questionnaire at the beginning of this chapter is designed to help you determine whether this is the case. If you answered "yes" to many of the questions above, it is possible that sleep deprivation is impairing your cognitive ability. This chapter will provide you with information on the causes and symptoms of chronic insomnia, and help you understand what you can do to treat it. By preventing or alleviating chronic insomnia, you maybe able to help prevent against memory loss and cognitive decline. Let's first explore the major types of insomnia and their causes.

TYPES OF INSOMNIA

In categorizing insomnia, doctors generally look at the length of its duration. There are two main forms of insomnia: acute and chronic. *Acute insomnia* occurs over a relatively brief period of time. Trouble sleeping can last for a few days (a condition called *transient insomnia*), or for up to three weeks (a condition called *short-term insomnia*). Acute insomnia is a temporary problem, caused by travel, environmental factors, a traumatic event, or stress at work or at home.

By contrast, *chronic* or *long-term insomnia* lasts for a month or more. There are two primary types of chronic insomnia. Chronic insomnia is often the result of a more deep-seated physiological problem, including certain medical conditions, pharmaceutical drug use, or sleep disorders. Because this type of chronic insomnia can essentially be considered a symptom of a larger medical issue, it is called *secondary insomnia*. *Primary insomnia* occurs when the insomnia is not related to an underlying illness, but is often a prolonged psychological reaction to a stressful situation or trauma.

Many cases of acute insomnia can be resolved simply by removing or mitigating the effects of the immediate cause of the sleep loss, or by improving the practices and habits that surround your normal sleep routine. Chapter 10 outlines the lifestyle changes you can make in order to reduce stress and generally attain better sleep.

Because chronic insomnia is a more complex condition with significant and potentially long-lasting effects on your memory, its causes and treatment options are discussed at length here.

SYMPTOMS OF CHRONIC INSOMNIA

The symptoms of chronic insomnia are largely the same as those of acute insomnia, with the important distinction being that in chronic insomnia, the symptoms endure for a much longer period of time. Among others, symptoms can include:

- Fatigue

- Gastrointestinal distress

- Impaired performance throughout the day

- Mood changes (irritability, depression, anxiety)

- Tension headaches

- Trouble falling asleep at night (thirty minutes or longer to fall asleep)

- Trouble staying asleep at night (waking up frequently)

- Trouble staying awake during the day

- Waking up too early in the morning

CAUSES OF CHRONIC INSOMNIA

- Arthritis
- Attention deficit hyperactivity disorder
- Bipolar disorder
- Chronic anxiety or depression
- Chronic fatigue syndrome
- Chronic pain or fibromyalgia
- Disruptions to circadian rhythms (twenty-four hour sleep-wake cycle)
- Drug withdrawal

- Fear of insomnia
- Gastrointestinal disorders (including heartburn)
- Gluten intolerance
- Hormonal imbalance
- Neurotransmitter imbalance
- Post-traumatic stress disorder
- Restless leg syndrome
- Sleep apnea
- Thyroid disorders

Another significant source of chronic insomnia is the use of certain pharmaceutical drugs, including, but not limited to:

- Antiarrhythmics
- Anticonvulsants
- Antihistamines
- Appetite suppressants
- Benzodiazepines
- Beta blockers
- Bronchodilators
- Caffeine
- Carbidopa-levodopa (Sinemet)
- Diuretics
- Decongestants
- Marijuana or other recreational drugs

- Monoamine oxidase inhibitors
- Oral contraceptives
- Pseudoephedrine
- Selective serotonin reuptake inhibitors (SSRIs)
- Sedatives
- Statins
- Steroids
- Sympathomimetics
- Tetrahydrozoline
- Thyroid medication
- Tricyclic antidepressants

RISK FACTORS

Certain factors contribute to your risk of developing chronic insomnia:

- **Age**. People over the age of sixty are more prone to insomnia, due to changes in sleep patterns brought about by shifting hormone levels.

- **Frequent long-distance travel**. People who change time zones frequently disrupt their natural sleep-wake cycles.

- **Gender**. Women are more likely than men to develop insomnia.

- **Mental status**. People who suffer from depression or an emotional trauma are at greater risk.

- **Night shifts**. People who work at night disrupt their natural sleep-wake cycles.

- **Sedentary lifestyle**. People who are physically inactive are at greater risk.

- **Stress level**. People who suffer chronic stress or an intense emotional disturbance are at greater risk.

DIAGNOSING CHRONIC INSOMNIA

If you suspect that you suffer from chronic insomnia, your doctor will generally begin by giving you a questionnaire similar to the one at the beginning of this chapter. The purpose of the questionnaire is to establish potential sources of the insomnia, and to assess its intensity and duration. Your physician may also recommend that you keep a *sleep diary*, or a written record of sleep habits over a week or two: what times you went to bed and woke up, how long it took to fall asleep, how frequently you woke up during the night, etc. Medical tests can also be prescribed in order to determine whether your insomnia is actually a symptom of an underlying condition such as a thyroid disorder or hormonal imbalance.

If the source of your insomnia cannot be easily pinpointed, or if your insomnia fails to respond to treatment, you may be asked to complete an overnight sleep study at a sleep disorder center or lab. There, while you sleep, you will undergo a polysomnogram (PSG), a test that measures vital signs, including brain activity, eye movement, heart rate, blood pressure, and blood oxygen levels. If your doctor suspects that your insomnia is the result of sleep apnea, a common disorder in which your breathing is disrupted during sleep, your breathing may alternatively be monitored using a continuous positive airway pressure (CPAP) machine.

TREATMENT OPTIONS FOR CHRONIC INSOMNIA

Any treatment regimen for chronic insomnia should begin with an evaluation and, if necessary, alteration of sleep hygiene. By changing your habits—using your bedroom only for sleeping, eliminating or reducing stressors, avoiding both stimulants and depressants, and getting regular exercise, for example—you may be able to improve the quality and quantity of your sleep, and thus also your memory and focus. You will find a more extensive guide to proper sleep habits in Chapter 10.

For most cases of chronic insomnia, however, it will not be enough to simply change your sleep habits. Fortunately, there are now a wide variety of options available to people who suffer from chronic insomnia.

Behavioral Therapy

Behavioral therapy seeks to address the sources of insomnia by changing sleep-related behaviors and habits. Evidence suggests that behavioral therapy can be just as effective as medication in remedying or preventing insomnia—if not more so! This is because, unlike medications, behavioral therapy treats the cause of insomnia, not the symptoms. There are several different forms of behavioral therapy that can be used to treat insomnia.

Cognitive-Behavioral Therapy

Cognitive-behavioral therapy (CBT) uses a variety of techniques to identify and control negative thoughts and beliefs about sleep. For many people, insomnia becomes a source of worry or anxiety in and of itself; sometimes the fear that you will be unable to sleep becomes the very reason you can't. Either in personal or group sessions, a therapist will help you isolate and analyze the false or negative thoughts that prevent you from getting to sleep. By recognizing and rejecting these thoughts, cognitive-behavioral theorists reason, you will be able to eliminate the source of much insomnia. For best results, CBT is often used in conjunction with other behavioral techniques, such as sleep restriction or stimulus control.

Paradoxical Intention Therapy

Like cognitive-behavioral therapy, paradoxical intention therapy is used for patients whose insomnia is the result of anxiety over the inability to sleep. This form of therapy asserts that since worrying about sleep makes you unable to sleep, you must eliminate this worry by avoiding any attempt to fall asleep. Instead, you are told to get into bed and stay awake. By forcing yourself to undergo the experience that you fear most—lying awake in bed—you make it less scary, thus preventing insomnia by reducing any "performance anxiety" associated with falling asleep.

Relaxation Training and Biofeedback

Relaxation training teaches you to more quickly initiate sleep by employing imagery methods, special breathing techniques, or by progressively tensing and relaxing different muscle groups from the feet on up to the face. Sometimes relaxation training is done in coordination with biofeedback, in which certain vital signs (blood pressure, muscle tension, electrical activity in the brain) are monitored. The idea is that by watching the changes in your vital signs, you will learn to recognize the physiological patterns and tendencies that are generated as you attempt to relax, so that you will be better able to duplicate the process of relaxation at home, in bed.

Sleep Restriction Therapy

Sleep restriction aims to improve insomnia by recalibrating your homeostatic sleep drive, or your biological imperative to sleep. This it does by limiting the amount of time you spend in bed to the approximate number of hours you are normally able to sleep. Thus, if on average you sleep five hours a night, you will spend just five hours in bed—regardless of the amount of time you actually end up sleeping during that period. The first few weeks of this therapy can be tough, as you may be getting far less sleep than you are used to getting. Eventually, however, the sleep loss will make you tired enough that you fall asleep more quickly, getting the most out of the limited time you actually spend in bed. After you have optimized your time in bed, you can then begin to gradually increase your time allotment, leading to more and better sleep.

Stimulus Control Therapy

Stimulus control therapy has proven to be one of the most effective behavioral therapies commonly used to treat insomnia. In stimulus control therapy, patients learn to associate the bed and bedroom (the "cue" or stimulus) with sleep and sex only. By strengthening this association, patients find it easier to fall asleep, both initially and after waking in the middle of the night. Some of the strategies used to reinforce stimulus control include: going to bed only when already sleepy, getting up and leaving the bedroom if sleep doesn't arrive within fifteen minutes, avoiding naps, and maintaining a relatively strict sleep schedule.

MEDICATIONS

There is a wide range of medications used to treat insomnia. Some are available by prescription only, while others can be purchased over the counter. While effective in the short term, particularly if the insomnia is the result of a temporary source of stress, care must be used when using any medication that induces sleep. Side effects, including impaired thinking, sleep walking or sleep eating, agitation, and poor balance, are common, particularly in adults over the age of sixty. In addition, certain prescription sleep medications can be habit-forming, making it harder to sleep without the use of these drugs.

Because of these risks, most doctors recommend that their patients use sleep aids infrequently, or for short periods only. If you are considering using a medication to treat your insomnia, talk to your doctor so that you are fully aware of the effects that such a regimen might have on your personal medical status.

Prescription Medications

According to a recent study, about 13 percent of all American adults have used a prescription medication to relieve the symptoms of insomnia in the past year, with nearly two percent using a medication on any given day. In total, almost 100 million prescriptions for medications to aid with sleep are written each year. These medications include drugs expressly formulated to initiate and maintain sleep, including:

- Alprazolam (Xanax)
- Clonazepam (Klonopin)
- Eszopiclone (Lunesta)
- Flurazepam (Dalmane)
- Lorazepam (Ativan)

- Ramelteon (Rozerem)
- Triazolam (Halcion)
- Zaleplon (Sonata)
- Zolpidem (Ambien)

In addition, antidepressants are often prescribed, both to treat cases of secondary insomnia that are caused by depression, and also to be exploited for their sedative effects in cases of primary insomnia. Antidepressants commonly prescribed to treat insomnia include:

- Amitriptyline (Elavil)
- Doxepin (Silenor)
- Mirtazapine (Remeron)

- Trazodone (Desyrel)
- Trimipramine (Surmontil)

Nonprescription Medications

Most drugstores carry over-the-counter sleep aids. These nonprescription medications usually include an antihistamine, often diphenhydramine (Benadryl) or doxylamine (Unison). Sometimes the antihistamine is combined with a pain reliever, as in Tylenol PM—these combination sleep aids can be particularly helpful for those whose insomnia is the result of chronic pain, arthritis, or fibromyalgia.

Hormone Therapy

As explained in Chapter 4, hormones play important roles in regulating every aspect of your health—and sleep is no exception. Different hormones, including DHEA, cortisol, thyroid hormones, sex hormones, and growth hormone promote good sleep in both men and women. When these hormones get out of balance, as in menopause or andropause, chronic insomnia can often be the result. Sustaining an appropriate balance of these hormones is thus very important when attempting to treat chronic insomnia.

By far the most influential hormone, at least where sleep is concerned, is melatonin. Melatonin is a key ingredient that helps control your circadian rhythms, the twenty-four hour cycles that, among other tasks, govern when you sleep and wake (sometimes referred to as the "sleep-wake cycle"). Specifically, melatonin is the hormone that tells your body when to go to sleep, with levels peaking shortly before you go to bed at night. Studies have shown that supplementing with melatonin can help both induce and maintain sleep, keeping you from waking up during the night. Melatonin can also be used to remedy insomnia that is the result of travel to a different time zone; when taken as directed, melatonin essentially resets your circadian rhythms.

In order to see if melatonin supplementation will help your insomnia, consult with a metabolic or anti-aging specialist, who will order a test to see if your melatonin levels are low. If they are, your doctor may advise you to begin supplementing with as little as 0.5 milligrams of melatonin, taken half an hour to an hour before bedtime—though doses of 1 to 3 milligrams may be more effective. You do not want to take melatonin if you do not need it, since too much melatonin will lower your levels of serotonin and can cause depression. Furthermore, high doses of melatonin may actually cause insomnia.

Neurotransmitter Therapy

Your sleep-wake cycle is regulated not only by hormones, but also by neurotransmitters—particularly serotonin, dopamine, norepinephrine, and acetylcholine, your main memory neurotransmitter. Of all the neurotransmitters, serotonin is perhaps the most important for good sleep: it helps initiate the first four stages of sleep (non-REM sleep, the kind that is most important for the consolidation of memories) and also promotes wakefulness. Accordingly, it is important to keep your levels of this neurotransmitter high by taking supplements that boost serotonin production, including the amino acid tryptophan and its derivative, 5-hydroxytryptophan (5-HTP). Clinical studies show that tryptophan is useful for people who have trouble getting to sleep, whereas 5-HTP is preferred for people who have trouble staying asleep.

Alternatively, you can take the amino acid L-theanine, which is derived from green tea. L-theanine increases both serotonin and dopamine production, and is good for reducing "mind chatter"—the mental restlessness that prevents some people from falling asleep easily. It should be taken twice a day for best results.

All three amino acid supplements have significant advantages over pharmaceutical treatments for insomnia: while effective for treating insomnia, they do not change the normal sleep process, and they do not cause withdrawal symptoms. For dosage and instructions, see the table on page 95.

Dietary Supplements

The following is a comprehensive list of supplements that may help relieve your insomnia.

Supplement	Dosage	Considerations
California Poppy (*Eschscholzia californica*)	Use as directed.	Extract concentrations vary from brand to brand; for this reason, it is best to follow dosage instructions as indicated on label.
Chamomile	Drink as a tea three to four times daily.	Do not use in conjunction with other sedatives, including alcohol. Should not be taken with anticoagulants or by anyone whose blood does not clot easily.
5-hydroxytryp-tophan (5-HTP)	50 to 300 mg daily.	Can be taken with magnesium for increased effectiveness. May interfere with antidepressants. Should not be taken with medications for Parkinson's disease. Consult with your doctor before taking if you have diabetes, high blood pressure, heart disease, or an autoimmune disorder.
Hops	Use as directed.	Extract concentrations vary from brand to brand; for this reason, it is best to follow dosage instructions as indicated on label.
Lavender	Use as directed.	Extract concentrations vary from brand to brand; for this reason, it is best to follow dosage instructions as indicated on label.
Lemon balm	Use as directed.	Do not take if you have glaucoma.
L-theanine	100 to 200 mg, taken in the morning and evening.	Extract concentrations vary from brand to brand; for this reason, it is best to follow dosage instructions as indicated on label.
Magnesium	400 to 600 mg daily.	May cause loose stools.
Magnolia officinalis	Use as directed.	Extract concentrations vary from brand to brand; for this reason, it is best to follow dosage instructions as indicated on label.
Melatonin	0.5 to 3 mg daily.	High doses may cause dizziness, headaches, insomnia, or depression. May amplify the effects of medications that lower blood pressure, or increase blood sugar levels in some diabetics.
Passionflower	Use as directed.	High doses may cause irregular heartbeat (arrhythmia). May interfere with monoamine oxidase (MAO) inhibitors.
Tryptophan	2,000 mg daily.	Avoid protein intake just before use. Can be taken with vitamin B_6, B_3, or magnesium for maximum effectiveness. May interfere with selective serotonin reuptake inhibitors (SSRIs) or monoamine oxidase (MAO) inhibitors.

Supplement	Dosage	Considerations
Valerian (*Valeriana officinalis*)	Use as directed.	Should be taken with vitamin B_6, B_3, or magnesium for maximum effectiveness. Can cause headaches, dizziness, restlessness, heart palpitations, or gastrointestinal disturbances. Should not be taken by women who are pregnant or nursing.
Vitamin B_1 (thiamine)	10 to 100 mg daily	High doses may deplete your body of vitamin B_6 (pyridoxine) and magnesium.
Vitamin B_3 (niacinamide)	50 to 3,000 mg daily	Sedative effects may be amplified by simultaneously taking L-tryptophan. Can cause skin flushing, sensations of heat, stomach problems, or dry skin. Consult with your doctor if taking more than 100 mg daily; higher doses can cause liver damage, peptic ulcers, or glucose intolerance. Should not be taken by those who suffer from liver disease, or at the same time as other B-complex vitamins.
Vitamin B_{12} (cobalamin)	800 to 1,000 mcg daily	May cause diarrhea, blood clots, itching, or allergic reactions. Consult with your healthcare provider before using if you have high blood pressure or other forms of heart disease.
Ziziphus spinosa	Use as directed.	Extract concentrations vary from brand to brand; for this reason, it is best to follow dosage instructions as indicated on label.

Other Treatments

Due to the prevalence of insomnia in society today, new treatment options are constantly being developed. Microcurrent therapy, homeopathy, magnetic therapy, yoga, and acupuncture have all been shown to be helpful in relieving insomnia. Stress management, discussed in Chapter 11, can have an enormous effect on your sleep capacity. In addition, by adopting many of the practices discussed in Chapter 10, you may be able to attain noticeable improvements in your sleep. Exercise, discussed in Chapter 8, can also help reduce and even prevent sleep disorders.

CONCLUSION

Because sleep plays such an important role in the consolidation of memories, prolonged sleep deprivation or chronic insomnia can seriously weaken your recall and ability to focus. Having read this chapter, you now know how to recognize the risk factors, causes, and symptoms of insomnia, and thus can determine whether this condition is affecting you or your loved ones. By understanding that memory loss can be an effect of chronic insomnia, you will be better equipped to treat the problem at the source, using the treatment options detailed above or in Chapter 10.

7

Dementia

Dementia is an umbrella term that encompasses the most severe forms of memory loss and cognitive decline. Generally speaking, dementia results from the widespread death or malfunction of your neurons (brain cells), but the direct cause of this damage to your brain varies from condition to condition. Dementia is *not* a natural consequence of aging, but rather the result of external conditions or disease processes that occur more frequently among older populations. Unlike the other types of memory loss described in Chapter 1, most forms of dementia are both unpreventable and nonreversible. In other words, at this time, dementia can be neither avoided nor cured.

This chapter explores the most common forms and causes of dementia, enabling you to recognize specific conditions that may affect yourself or others. This awareness can be critical to your health and wellbeing, since in most cases the exact cause of dementia can only be positively confirmed with a brain autopsy after death. With this foundation of knowledge established, the chapter then provides an overview of the treatment options available for those suffering from these extreme forms of memory loss. While there is no known remedy for most forms of dementia, there are many ways to slow its advancement, so that you and your loved ones can live long, mindful lives.

ALZHEIMER'S DISEASE (AD)

Alzheimer's disease (AD) is a progressive or neurodegenerative form of dementia, meaning that it is characterized by the gradual deterioration and destruction of your brain cells. Over time, an Alzheimer's patient's entire brain shrinks or atrophies, affecting all aspects of cognition and resulting in profound memory loss. Although early-onset Alzheimer's (defined as Alzheimer's disease that has begun before the age of sixty) is possible as the result of genetic factors, Alzheimer's disease is primarily late-onset, manifesting after the age of sixty. Death from AD, or from a condition to which AD has contributed, can occur from three to ten years after initial diagnosis, depending on the rate at which the disease advances and the age of the patient who is suffering.

Alzheimer's disease is the most common cause of dementia, accounting for an estimated 60 to 80 percent of all dementia cases. In the United States, about 5.2 million Americans suffer from this disease; by 2050, this number could triple to nearly 14 million. It is the sixth leading cause of death amongst individuals of all ages and the fifth leading cause of death for people over the age of 65.

The cost of Alzheimer's disease is staggering, and is likely to increase even more as baby boomers age. People with AD and other forms of dementia have three times as many hospital visits each year as do individuals with no dementia; Alzheimer's patients are also likely to require more frequent home health care visits and skilled nursing facility stays. In addition, due to their inability to care for themselves, Alzheimer's patients are twice as likely as normal individuals to need long-term nonmedical paid home care. Between long-term care, health care, and hospice costs, it is estimated that about $203 billion is spent on Alzheimer's patients each year—and that figure could rise to $1.2 trillion by 2050.

Symptoms

Because Alzheimer's is a progressive condition, damage to the cerebrum and hippocampus develops over a period of years, and symptoms may not appear until long after the disease has begun to develop. Typically, patients start to notice significant symptoms after the age of sixty; as time passes, these symptoms worsen and become more detrimental to the individual's overall quality of life. Episodic memory is the first to be affected, followed by short-term, semantic, and procedural memory (see pages 11 to 12). As the disease advances, nearly all brain functions are affected; eventually, even physical capabilities like swallowing or bowel control can become impaired.

Alzheimer's disease presents itself in a variety of ways.

- Confusion with time or place
- Decline in comprehension of spatial relationships
- Delusions
- Difficulty learning
- Difficulty multitasking
- Disorientation
- Impaired judgment
- Inability to plan or strategize

- Memory loss that interferes with daily functioning
- Mental or emotional disorders (anxiety, depression, paranoia)
- Personality changes
- Social withdrawal
- Trouble communicating (difficulty finding the right words, inability to read/write)

Causes

Despite a wealth of research on the subject, scientists are still unsure as to the cause or causes of Alzheimer's disease. Currently, only one cause of Alzheimer's disease has been positively identified—a set of deterministic genetic mutations that, when inherited, create a near certainty that the bearer will develop Alzheimer's disease before the age of sixty. These gene variants—amyloid precursor protein (APP), presenilin-1 (PS-1) and presenilin-2 (PS-2)—affect your ability to process a protein called amyloid, leading to large and damaging deposits of this substance in your brain. Cases of these genetic mutations are very rare, however—less than five percent of Alzheimer's patients are diagnosed with the resulting *dominantly inherited Alzheimer's disease.*

So what causes Alzheimer's disease in the general population? What makes patients' brain cells die at such an elevated rate? In seeking the source of the problem, researchers most frequently look at the "hallmark" brain abnormalities and biochemical conditions that characterize the brains of Alzheimer's patients. Although it is unclear whether these abnormalities or conditions are really the causes of neuron death, or are themselves the result of an underlying problem, several theories have emerged.

Beta-Amyloid Plaque Theory

One of the most prominent theories of Alzheimer's disease places the blame on the disease's characteristic proliferation of beta-amyloid plaques—sticky clumps of protein that block synapses and prevent electrical signals from traveling between neurons in the brain. When your neurons are thus unable to perform their most essential function, they die, leading to the cognitive decline and memory loss that we associate with Alzheimer's disease.

Most people have a certain volume of these plaques, but various factors seem to encourage more widespread plaque growth and neuron death, including the genetic mutations discussed above. While this theory has become increasingly popular over the last few decades, recent studies indicate that the plaques are more likely to be the byproduct, not the cause, of the true problem. At best, research is inconclusive; more work must be done to determine the exact role of beta-amyloid protein in Alzheimer's disease.

Neurotransmitters and Cognitive Decline

Hormones aren't the only chemicals that affect your brain. Research increasingly shows that neurotransmitter imbalances can also impair your memory and mental acuity. As you'll remember, neurotransmitters are the chemicals that allow your brain cells (neurons) to communicate with each other. Neurotransmitters transport messages—encoded as electrical signals—at lightning speeds across the synapses between your neurons, enabling all forms of cognitive function. Every thought and feeling that you have, and every action and reaction that you perform is made possible by neurotransmission.

There are four neurotransmitters that are heavily linked to memory formation, storage, and retrieval: acetylcholine, dopamine, serotonin, and glutamate. Acetylcholine is your main memory neurotransmitter, and is critical to issues of attention and arousal as well. Dopamine is a neurotransmitter that is heavily associated with the processing of pleasure and pain, and also with concentration, problem-solving, and both working and long-term memory (see pages 10 to 11). Serotonin is best known for regulating mood, anxiety, and appetite, but also seems to play an important role in cognition. Finally, the neurotransmitter glutamate can be toxic to your brain cells in large volumes, but when possessed in appropriate amounts, it is integral to learning and memory formation.

In addition to their specific roles in supporting cognition, neuro-

Cholinergic Theory

As you'll remember from Chapter 1, brain levels of neurotransmitters—the chemicals that help conduct electrical signals between your neurons—naturally decrease as you age. In Alzheimer's disease, levels of certain neurotransmitters associated with memory and cognitive performance have been shown to be especially low. The cholinergic theory suggests that Alzheimer's disease begins with a decline in the production of acetylcholine, your brain's main memory neurotransmitter (see inset on page 102). The problem with this theory is that Alzheimer's patients demonstrate very low levels of this neurotransmitter throughout the progression of the disease process; low acetylcholine is thus less likely to *cause* Alzheimer's disease and more likely to be a manifestation of a larg-

transmitters also indirectly shape memory, as they govern other factors and processes that can potentially influence cognitive function, including mood, stress, toxin removal, energy availability, and cardiovascular health. Critically, neurotransmitters play an important role in helping your body break down homocysteine, an amino acid that is associated not only with a higher risk of heart disease (itself a risk factor for cognitive decline) but also with a higher risk of Alzheimer's disease.

It is important to note that neurotransmitters form a complex web with hormones; the two substances interact with and modulate each other. In some cases, hormones can even act as neurotransmitters, indicating that the different chemical systems of the body are far more integrated than previously thought. More research must be done to investigate the ways that these powerful chemicals work together to affect the brain and cognitive decline.

Because neurotransmitters are essential to thought and memory, low levels or imbalances of these vital substances can result in significant deficits in your ability to focus and remember. Your neurotransmitter levels will naturally decline somewhat as you age, but abnormally low levels of the neurotransmitters acetylcholine and serotonin are a hallmark of Alzheimer's disease. Consult with a metabolic or anti-aging specialist to have your neurotransmitter levels measured; your doctor may recommend that you eat certain foods or add special supplements to your diet in order to rectify any neurotransmitter deficiencies that you might have.

er underlying problem. In addition, acetylcholine isn't the only neuro-transmitter to be depleted; levels of serotonin are also abnormally low in Alzheimer's patients. Even if acetylcholine is not the direct cause of Alzheimer's disease, more research needs to be done to explore the complex roles of neurotransmitters in cognitive decline.

Tau Theory

Another characteristic element of Alzheimer's disease is the presence of neurofibrillary (tau) tangles. Inside normal neurons, tau protein strands help maintain cell integrity and assist in the transport of nutrients within the cell. Inside the neurons of people with Alzheimer's disease, these strands form snarls, preventing the brain cells from functioning and transporting nutrients, and eventually instigating their death. Scientists are currently investigating why these tau proteins thus fold improperly, believing the cause may hold the key to Alzheimer's disease.

Inflammation Theory

Recently, scientists have suggested that inflammation is the underlying disease process that explains why beta-amyloid plaques accumulate—and thus why Alzheimer's disease develops. When inflammation occurs (see Chapter 5), your brain undergoes certain chemical changes that result in the increased production and altered shape of amyloid proteins. Inflammation may also play a role in instigating excess activity in your brain's immune cells—the glial cells (see page 6)—and may be directly responsible for the destruction or toxicity of neurons.

Oxidative Stress Theory

Studies consistently demonstrate the presence of excessive oxidation (free radical production) in the brains of Alzheimer's patients. While free radicals are essential to the metabolism of glucose, allowing your brain to receive the energy it needs to function properly, too many free radicals—as a result of injury, infection, inflammation, or heavy metal accumulation—can cause toxicity and brain cell death.

Metal Metabolism Theories

Various studies have suggested that imbalances of trace minerals, including mercury, copper and iron, can cause Alzheimer's disease. Copper and iron are sources of free radicals in the brain; excess volumes of these metals can thus raise oxidative stress and inflammation (see above). In addition, high levels of copper can increase the development of beta-amyloid plaques, or possibly prevent their removal. At the same time, other studies have indicated that copper might protect against Alzheimer's disease. Like many aspects of human biochemistry, too much or too little of any substance can destroy the delicate balance that is necessary for the body to function optimally.

Because a protein called metallothionein can help regulate copper and zinc levels, and thus oxidative stress and inflammation, scientists are looking into the possibility of using it as a treatment for Alzheimer's disease.

Risk Factors

Although the causes of Alzheimer's disease are not well understood, comparatively more is known about the factors that can increase the likelihood that a person will develop this condition. Among others, significant risk factors include:

- **Age.** Age is the single greatest risk factor in Alzheimer's disease. According to the Alzheimer's Association, the likelihood of developing Alzheimer's disease doubles about every five years after the age of sixty-five; by age eighty-five, risk approximates nearly fifty percent.

- **Family history.** Those with a parent or sibling with Alzheimer's disease are more likely to develop Alzheimer's. The more close relatives with Alzheimer's, the greater the risk.

- **Genetics.** In addition to the deterministic gene mutations mentioned above, the presence of the mutation apolipoprotein-e4 (APOE-e4) indicates a higher risk of developing Alzheimer's disease.

- **Mild Cognitive Impairment.** See page 14.

- **Cardiovascular disease.** See Chapter 2.

- **Traumatic Brain Injury (TBI).**

- **Down's syndrome.**

- **Diabetes and insulin resistance.** See Chapter 4.

- **Low education attainment.**

- **Poor social and cognitive engagement.**

Other possible risk factors include:

- **Sex.** Women are more likely than men to develop Alzheimer's disease, although that may be simply because they also tend to live longer.

- **Alcohol and drug abuse**

- **Heavy metal exposure**

- **Exposure to industrial solvents and pesticides**

- **Advanced maternal age**

- **Infection**

- **Thyroid disease**

Diagnosis

There is no specific test to determine whether a person has Alzheimer's disease. If Alzheimer's disease is suspected, your doctor will carry out a thorough medical evaluation in order to rule out other types and causes of memory loss. Tests may include:

- **Review of medical history.**

- **Physical and neurological exam.** To test reflexes, coordination, balance, muscle tone and strength, and sensory processing.

- **Neuropsychological tests.** To assess different categories of cognitive function; different skills/abilities are affected by different forms of dementia.

- **Mental status testing.** To assess memory, general thinking skills.

- **Lab tests.** To rule out thyroid disorders or nutritional deficiencies that may be causing memory loss.

- **Brain imaging.** Computerized tomography (CT) scans, magnetic resonance imaging (MRI), positron emission tomography (PET) scans, or single photon emission computed tomography (SPECT) might be used to locate or identify brain abnormalities caused not by Alzheimer's disease, but rather by strokes, traumas, or tumors.

VASCULAR DEMENTIA (VAD)

Vascular dementia (VaD), sometimes called multi-infarct or post-stroke dementia, is the second most common form of dementia in the United

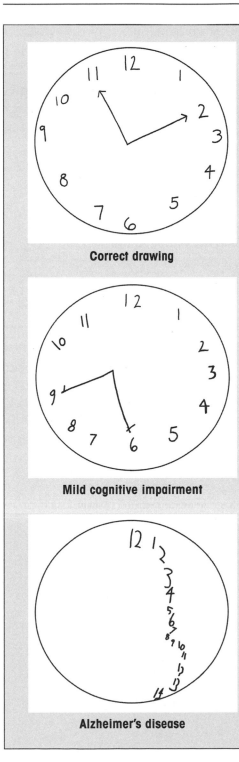

Correct drawing

Mild cognitive impairment

Alzheimer's disease

The Clock Drawing Test

One of the most useful diagnostic tools used by doctors to screen for cognitive impairment and dementia is the clock drawing test. In it, a patient is asked to either draw the face of a clock from memory (circle, numbers), or to draw numbers representing a clock face on a predrawn circle.

Even in the earliest stages of dementia, patients can have trouble with the visual organization of space, and will thus have difficulty completing the task—numbers may be drawn out of order or in the wrong place (or outside the circle), the numbers may not be spaced adequately, or they may not be written correctly at all.

Scoring methods vary, but points are generally awarded for the accuracy of the depiction.

States, accounting for 20 to 30 percent of all dementia cases. It is defined as a decline in thinking skills and memory caused by interrupted blood flow to the brain, often as the result of a stroke or series of strokes. In order to function properly, your brain requires a large volume of oxygen and nutrients, which it receives through an extensive network of blood vessels. When these blood vessels are blocked or damaged—as by a stroke or other forms of cardiovascular disease—your brain cells are deprived of the substances they need, and quickly begin to die, initiating memory loss and other cognitive dysfunction.

Unlike the other major forms of dementia, vascular dementia is at least partially preventable; by controlling the risk factors that contribute to heart disease, you can significantly reduce the likelihood that you will ever suffer from this disease. For more information, see Chapter 2.

Symptoms

Symptoms of vascular dementia vary according to the area of the brain affected by the loss of blood flow and the severity of the damage, but tend to manifest initially in the form of confusion and impaired judgment; memory loss is common but not necessarily present. Cognitive decline can appear suddenly after a major stroke, or it can develop more gradually as damage accumulates from atherosclerosis (narrowing or hardening of the arteries) or a series of smaller strokes.

Principal symptoms include:

- Confusion
- Disorientation

- Loss of vision
- Trouble communicating

Other common symptoms include:

- Apathy
- Attention deficits
- Depression
- Impaired judgment
- Impaired motor function
- Impaired problem-solving

- Inability to plan or strategize
- Lack of coordination or balance; unsteady gait
- Memory loss
- Night wandering
- Restlessness

Causes

Vascular dementia is usually caused by a stroke or a series of strokes. A stroke, or infarction, occurs any time blood flow to your brain is interrupted. There are two types of strokes. Ischemic strokes are the most common, and are defined as strokes that severely reduce the volume of blood supplied to your brain. They take place when your brain arteries become severely narrowed by plaque (fatty deposits) or blocked by a blood clot. Hemorrhagic strokes are less common, and take place when a blood vessel in your brain ruptures (bursts) or leaks onto the surface of the brain, or into the brain itself, thus depriving your brain cells of the nutrients and oxygen they need.

Vascular dementia can also be caused by cardiovascular conditions that bring about the gradual deterioration of blood vessels in the brain, as by high blood pressure, atherosclerosis (hardened or narrowed arteries), or certain heart infections.

Risk Factors

As with most forms of dementia, age is the greatest single risk factor for vascular dementia. Although rarely seen in patients under the age of sixty-five, vascular dementia is more common and more likely in older populations.

Other risk factors for vascular dementia tend to mirror those of heart disease, since vascular dementia can in some ways be considered the byproduct of a cardiovascular condition. These risk factors include:

- Atherosclerosis (hardening or narrowing of the arteries)
- Atrial fibrillation (a type of arrhythmia)
- Diabetes
- High cholesterol
- High blood pressure
- History of cardiovascular disease
- Stroke

Diagnosis

Because the symptoms of vascular dementia sometimes appear gradually and can mimic or even coexist with those of Alzheimer's disease, vascular dementia sometimes goes undiagnosed or misdiagnosed. As with most forms of dementia, there is no single test to determine whether a patient has vascular dementia. Vascular dementia is usually diagnosed in response to a patient's medical history or evidence of stroke and other cardiovascular disease.

Often, doctors will order additional tests to clarify or confirm their diagnosis, or to rule out other sources of dementia. Exams include:

- **Blood tests.** To check for sources of dementia such as anemia, chronic infection, drug toxicity, low blood sugar, vitamin deficiencies, and thyroid disorders; and to evaluate risk factors such as cholesterol levels.

- **Blood pressure tests.**

- **Brain imaging.** Computerized tomography (CT) scans, magnetic resonance imaging (MRI), positron emission tomography (PET) scans, or single photon emission computed tomography (SPECT) might be used to locate or identify brain abnormalities caused by strokes, blood vessel diseases, traumas, or tumors.

- **Carotid ultrasound.** Uses soundwaves to identify and locate narrowing in carotid arteries (neck arteries that supply blood to the brain).

- **Mental status testing.** To assess memory, general thinking skills.

- **Neuropsychological tests.** To assess different categories of cognitive function; different skills/abilities are affected by different forms of dementia.

- **Physical and neurological exam.** To test reflexes, coordination, balance, muscle tone and strength, and sensory processing.

DEMENTIA WITH LEWY BODIES (DLB)

Dementia with Lewy bodies (DLB) is the third most common type of dementia, accounting for 10 to 25 percent of all cases and affecting an estimated 1.3 million Americans today. It is characterized by brain damage caused by Lewy bodies, protein clumps that are found in other neurodegenerative disorders, most notably Parkinson's disease and, to a lesser degree, Alzheimer's disease.

Symptoms

Because DLB has many pathological similarities to Parkinson's disease and Alzheimer's disease, it bears some resemblance to both diseases, entailing Alzheimer-like cognitive decline, and also Parkinsonian motor issues such as muscle rigidity and body tremors. Memory loss tends to be less prominent and pronounced in DLB than in other forms of dementia, but can be present. Instead, DLB is often identified by cognitive decline that affects executive functioning (the ability to analyze, strategize, or plan), and by the early manifestation of visual and auditory hallucinations.

Common symptoms include:

- Body tremors

- Delusions

- Depression

- Fluctuations in alertness in focus

- Impaired autonomic (automatic) functions (regulation of blood pressure, pulse, digestive processes)

- Impaired executive function (inability to analyze, strategize, or plan)

- Mild memory loss

- Rigidity

- Sleep disorders

- Trouble walking

- Visual and auditory hallucinations

Cause

Dementia with Lewy bodies seems to be caused by the accumulation of Lewy bodies—deposits of a certain type of protein called alpha synuclein—inside neurons in the cerebrum and the *substantia nigra*, a brain structure that controls movement. Scientists are not sure how exactly Lewy bodies contribute to brain cell death. Although there are obviously connections between DLB and both Alzheimer's disease and Parkinson's disease, further research is needed on this little-understood form of dementia.

Risk Factors

Because the cause of DLB has yet to be identified, risk factors also remain somewhat elusive for this form of dementia. Genetics do not seem to play a role; most DLB patients have no family history of the disease. As with other forms of dementia, age seems to be the primary risk factor; people over sixty are significantly more likely to develop DLB. There is also some evidence that DLB affects men more frequently than women.

Diagnosis

There is no single test to determine whether a patient has dementia with Lewy bodies. Generally, doctors look for dementia that is accompanied by at least two of the following symptoms:

- Fluctuating alertness and cognitive function

- Visual hallucinations

- Parkinsonian symptoms (muscle rigidity, trouble walking, tremors)

These features help distinguish DLB from other forms of dementia. In addition, your doctor may order any of the following tests:

- **Blood tests.** To check for sources of dementia such as anemia, chronic infection, drug toxicity, low blood sugar, vitamin deficiencies, and thyroid disorders; and to evaluate risk factors such as cholesterol levels.

- **Brain imaging.** Computerized tomography (CT) scans, magnetic resonance imaging (MRI), positron emission tomography (PET) scans, or single photon emission computed tomography (SPECT) might be used to locate or identify brain abnormalities caused not by DLB, but by strokes, blood vessel diseases, traumas, or tumors.

- **Electroencephalogram (EEG).** To rule out seizures or Creutzfeldt-Jakob disease, which also create fluctuations in alertness and cognitive ability.

- **Mental status testing.** To assess memory, general thinking skills.

- **Physical and neurological exam.** To test reflexes, coordination, balance, muscle tone and strength, and sensory processing.

- **Sleep evaluation.** To evaluate for the presence of sleep disorders, which are more common amongst patients with DLB than in patients with other forms of dementia.

FRONTOTEMPORAL DEMENTIA (FTD)

Frontotemporal dementia (FTD) describes a relatively rare group of disorders that primarily affect the frontal and temporal lobes. While it accounts for between 10 to 15 percent of all dementia cases, it is disproportionately common among younger patients, accounting for 20 to 50 percent of all dementia cases in people aged sixty-five or less.

Symptoms

Besides its early age of onset, FTD differs from other forms of dementia in that it is characterized by a progressive deterioration of behavior, language ability, and executive function (the ability to analyze, strategize, or plan); memory typically remains intact. There are three major types of FTD, each featuring a distinct set of symptoms.

Behavioral Variant FTD (bvFTD)

This form of FTD primarily affects behavior. Symptoms may include:

- Apathy

- Depression

- Deterioration in personal hygiene

- Hyperactivity

- Hypersexual behavior

- Inappropriate behavior

- Lack of judgment

- Loss of empathy and self-awareness

- Mood changes

- Overeating

- Personality changes

- Repetitive or compulsive behavior

Primary Progressive Aphasia (PPA)

PPA initially manifests as a deterioration in language skills, but can progress to behavioral problems such as those discussed above. There are two types of PPA:

- **Semantic dementia.** Patients speak fluently and correctly, but often with no regard to the actual conversation being conducted. They also tend to have difficulty recalling and using common words for specific objects: thus, a seagull may be referred to only as "bird," or a bird may be referred to only as "animal."

- **Progressive nonfluent aphasia.** Patients cannot speak fluently or correctly; they may be unable to understand written and spoken language.

FTD with Motor Neuron Disease (FTD/MND)

Patients with FTD/MND may have behavior and language problems as discussed above, but are also characterized by a number of motor difficulties, including:

- Clumsiness or difficulty with fine movements
- Difficulty swallowing
- Impaired coordination
- Muscle rigidity
- Muscle spasms

- Muscle weakness
- Shortness of breath (due to weakened breathing muscles)
- Tremors or twitches
- Unsteady gait

Causes

Scientists don't know what causes frontotemporal dementia, although many FTD cases are characterized by the presence of microscopic Pick bodies—tiny spheres of tau protein that accumulate inside your brain cells, causing them to lose function and die. Recently, studies have begun to find links between FTD and certain genetic mutations, although the extent of the associations—whether these mutations *cause* FTD or simply raise the likelihood of its development—is not well understood. In addition, it is unclear why the frontal and temporal lobes are specifically targeted. Researchers have hypothesized a connection between FTD/MND and amyotrophic lateral sclerosis (ALS, or Lou Gehrig's disease), as the two disorders seem to share certain genetic and physiological markers, including symptoms of motor dysfunction. More research is needed on these complex forms of dementia.

Risk Factors

Due to the lack of definitive data on the subject, the only known risk factor for FTD is a family history of the disease—although the majority of FTD patients (about 60 percent) have no family history of any neurodegenerative disease (including ALS or Alzheimer's).

Diagnosis

As with the other major forms of dementia, there is no single test to determine whether a person has FTD. Its early onset—patients are diagnosed at an average age of fifty-seven, thirteen years before the average Alzheimer's patient—is often the best clue in identifying this disease. Although FTD shares many symptoms with Alzheimer's disease, with which it is often confused, FTD can be distinguished from Alzheimer's by the prominence of speech and behavioral problems and the relative lack of memory loss.

To support a diagnosis of FTD, your doctor may also order tests, including:

- **Blood tests.** To check for sources of dementia such as anemia, chronic infection, drug toxicity, low blood sugar, vitamin deficiencies, and thyroid disorders; and to evaluate risk factors such as cholesterol levels.

- **Brain imaging.** Computerized tomography (CT) scans, magnetic resonance imaging (MRI), positron emission tomography (PET) scans, or single photon emission computed tomography (SPECT) might be used to locate or identify brain abnormalities caused not by FTD, but by strokes, blood vessel diseases, traumas, or tumors.

- **Mental status testing.** To assess memory, general thinking skills.

- **Neuropsychological tests.** To assess different categories of cognitive function; different skills/abilities are affected by different forms of dementia.

MIXED DEMENTIA

Mixed dementia is a medical state in which brain abnormalities associated with different forms of dementia are present at the same time. It most frequently refers to the coexistence of Alzheimer's disease and vascular dementia, but can also describe cases in which dementia with Lewy bodies coincides with Alzheimer's disease. Rarely, brain changes associated with Alzheimer's, vascular dementia, and DLB can all be present. Mixed dementia also acknowledges the fact that some forms of dementia are characterized by (and might stem from) the same brain abnormalities; for example, Lewy bodies can be found in both Alzheimer's and DLB patients.

Symptoms, causes, and risk factors of mixed dementia vary according to the types of dementia present. Because it is impossible to pinpoint the nature and variety of a patient's brain changes before an autopsy, patients with mixed dementia are often misdiagnosed as simply having the form of dementia that is responsible for the most prominent symptoms.

More research must be done into this recently identified problem, particularly as some scientists believe that the presence of multiple dementias can increase the rate and intensity at which patients develop symptoms.

OTHER TYPES OF DEMENTIA

In addition to the major types of dementia discussed above, dementia can be caused by various other diseases or conditions. Many of these causes cannot be avoided or prevented, including:

- Parkinson's disease

- Huntington's disease

- Creutzfeldt-Jakob disease

- Traumatic brain injury

- Normal pressure hydrocephalus (NPH)

Other causes of dementia are temporary or removable, meaning that they can potentially be prevented and even cured, including:

- Alcohol abuse

- Brain tumors

- Depression

- Dehydration

- Heavy metal toxicity

- Immune disorders

- Infections

- Metabolic and endocrine dysfunction

- Nutritional deficiencies

- Oxygen deprivation

- Reactions to medications

- Thyroid disorders

- Wernicke-Korsakoff syndrome

Several of these problems—and their solutions—have been discussed earlier in this book.

TREATMENT OPTIONS

While most forms of dementia cannot be prevented or cured, research shows that by managing some of the controllable (modifiable) risk factors associated with dementia, you may be able to delay the onset of these disorders or reduce the progression of their symptoms. In addition, certain medications may actually improve symptoms, at least temporarily.

Pharmaceutical Drugs

Currently, the United States Food and Drug Administration (FDA) has approved two categories of drugs for the treatment of Alzheimer's disease and certain other forms of dementia. Some of these drugs may also be effective in the treatment of vascular dementia. In addition to these drugs, which specifically treat cognitive decline, other medications may be prescribed to manage the depression, anxiety, sleep disorders, and behavioral disturbances that are also associated with dementia.

Cholinesterase Inhibitors

These drugs are used to treat Alzheimer's disease, DLB, vascular dementia, and mild cognitive impairment. They raise brain levels of the chemical acetylcholine, the main neurotransmitter responsible for the conduction of memory signals, potentially enhancing memory, attention, mood, and behavior. Unfortunately, less than half of all patients using cholinesterase inhibitors will see any improvement in their symptoms. In those that are helped by these drugs, the advancement of symptoms is delayed for only a short period of time—six to twelve months on average. Side effects are rare, but can include sleep disturbances, dehydration, rashes, slow heart rate, seizues, and gastrointestinal problems such as nausea, vomiting, diarrhea, and loss of appetite. Common cholinesterase inhibitors include donezepil (Aricept), rivastigimine (Exelon), and galantamine (Razadyne).

Memantine

Memantine (Namenda) regulates the levels of another neurotransmitter that aids in learning and memory, glutamate, and enhances the transmission of dopamine, which works in the hippocampus and the prefrontal cortex to aid in cognition. It has been shown to improve attention, apathy, alertness, and global functioning in patients with Alzheimer's disease, vascular dementia, DLB, and frontotemporal dementia. Like cholinesterase inhibitors, memantine has only a temporary window of effectiveness. Side effects are rare, but include dizziness, confusion, and drowsiness.

Lifestyle Changes

Certain lifestyle changes may improve symptoms and slow the progression of dementia.

Diet

Studies show that a diet that is low in fat and rich in fruits and vegetables—particularly cruciferous or green leafy vegetables (broccoli, kale, spinach)—may both prevent and reduce the symptoms associated with dementia. Foods that are high in omega-3 fatty acids, including fish such as salmon or mackerel, can also help improve symptoms. For more information, see Chapter 12.

Physical and Mental Activity

Regular physical activity has benefits for people of all ages and levels of memory loss. It may also help to improve mood and cognition by boosting neurotransmitter levels. Regular intellectual or mental activity is important, too; by challenging your mind with puzzles and word games, and by pursuing lifelong education, you can help maintain healthy neural connections and networks. For more information, see Chapters 8 and 9.

Lower Your Risk of Cardiovascular Disease

Cardiovascular disease is a major risk factor for the development of all kinds of dementia, but particularly vascular dementia. Keep your blood pressure and cholesterol levels low, don't smoke, and treat any existing heart conditions. For more information, see Chapter 2.

Supplements

While there is no supplement that can prevent or cure any form of dementia, there are many that can be used to treat and even improve some of the symptoms. For a more extensive discussion of these supplements, see Chapter 13.

CONCLUSION

As you have seen, dementia is a complex disease, and one that can have a devastating effect on your life and those of your loved ones. But even if you can't prevent or cure dementia altogether, there is still much that you can do to limit its impact on your life. The purpose of this book is to guide you in these matters, so that you are aware of all of the ways you can keep your mind sharp and avoid or restrict any cognitive decline.

PART II

THE SOLUTIONS

8

Physical Activity

Regular physical activity is essential to maintaining good health—not just for your body, but also your mind. Because of advances in technology and changes in working environments, Americans today live increasingly sedentary lives. Recent studies indicate that almost 80 percent of all Americans fail to meet the guidelines for physical activity recommended by the Centers for Disease Control and Prevention and the American College of Sports Medicine. Worse yet, physical inactivity causes nearly 1 in 10 premature deaths around the world each year, largely because it contributes to the risk of heart disease, type 2 diabetes, breast cancer, and colon cancer. One study estimates that if rates of physical inactivity were decreased worldwide by as little as 25 percent, more than a million deaths each year could be averted.

Clearly, lack of exercise is a problem with serious consequences for your wellbeing. Yet it is a problem that is easily solved! I was lucky to be able to meet fitness and nutrition expert Jack LaLanne before he passed away. When I asked him what I could do to learn to like exercise, he admitted that he didn't like exercising all that much himself—but he loved the results.

One of the great results of regular exercise is that your mind will stay sharp. Besides advancing your overall health and conditioning, physical activity has been shown to improve cognitive function and memory. In fact, according to *New York Times* health and science writer Gretchen Reynolds, some studies indicate that exercise potentially "does more to bolster thinking than thinking does." Research consistently shows that exercise is one of the most powerful tools available for enhancing mental capacity and even preventing memory loss. It reduces age-related memory impairment and protects against the development of dementia.

According to one study, middle-aged people who exercise are one-third as likely to get Alzheimer's disease in their seventies as those who did not exercise; even those who began exercising in their sixties saw dramatic improvements in their cognitive function, with risk of Alzheimer's reduced by as much as 50 percent.

The goal of this chapter is to provide you with the information you need to adopt or maintain a healthy exercise program. By getting the right amount of physical activity for your age and fitness level, you can help keep your mind as quick and accurate as it can possibly be. You may even increase your ability to think, remember, and reason!

First, let's examine what exercise is, and why it's so good for your brain.

WHAT IS PHYSICAL ACTIVITY? WHAT IS EXERCISE?

Physical activity is anything that gets your body moving. There are two main categories of physical activity: aerobic and anaerobic. *Aerobic activity*—often called endurance or cardiovascular activity—is any form of movement that increases your heart rate and requires additional intake of oxygen. By contrast, *anaerobic activity*—physical movement that helps build muscle mass—requires very little increase in oxygen intake, as it is typically shorter in duration and of higher intensity. Although aerobic activity is what organizations like the American College of Sports Medicine (ACSM) and the Centers for Disease Control and Prevention (CDC) are generally referring to when they give their recommendations for physical activity, both forms of movement are important to good brain and cognitive function. In fact, some research suggests that aerobic and anaerobic activity can engage and support different parts of the brain.

Physical activity can be incidental, as when you perform various household chores, including gardening, making beds, or vacuuming. Or it can take the form of exercise, which is defined as physical activity that is planned with the express purpose of boosting fitness and endurance; examples include running, biking, swimming, weight lifting, playing on a sports team, or even brisk walking. Regardless of how it's performed, physical activity is indispensable for good health and a sharp mind.

HOW DOES EXERCISE HELP YOUR MIND?

Most people are aware of the long-term physiological benefits of physical activity. Exercise boosts your energy levels, helps you control your weight, strengthens your muscles and bones, and decreases your risk of developing type 2 diabetes and cancers of the breast, colon, and prostate. On the most basic level, regular exercise enhances your general quality of life.

By contrast, fewer people are conscious of the cognitive benefits of aerobic exercise. This is a shame, for research increasingly and unanimously shows that physical activity has a powerful impact on your ability to think and recall. While studies agree that aerobic exercise —involving moderate physical activity—is the best way to help your mind, even nonaerobic exercise, like weight or resistance training, can provide benefits for your brain. Exercise affects your brain both directly and indirectly. As you have seen in previous chapters, exercise can indirectly influence your cognitive ability by helping to prevent or reduce inflammation, cardiovascular disease, stress, and insomnia—all factors that can impair your memory and mental acuity.

Exercise also plays a number of direct roles in supporting your brain and cognition. For one thing, it seems to stimulate the growth of brain cells and protect against brain cell death. You may remember from Chapter 1 that normal age-related memory impairment is linked in part to mild brain deterioration or shrinkage. Research has shown that exercise can help limit the extent to which your brain shrinks. Better still, exercise can even make your brain bulk up and grow bigger. One region that seems to respond especially well to exercise is the hippocampus—your brain's memory center—which is ordinarily quite vulnerable to the wear and tear of the aging process. In one trial involving 120 adults with an average age of sixty-seven and no evidence of dementia, subjects who adopted a moderate, thrice-weekly aerobic exercise program actually saw an increase in hippocampal volume over a one-year period, effectively reversing age-related decline by one to two years. Not surprisingly, this increase in hippocampal volume also seemed to produce improvements in certain types of memory performance.

Exercise not only creates new brain cells, but also helps produce and maintain their support systems. All these new brain cells require added nutrients and oxygen; to meet this demand, exercise actually seems to increase both the number of blood vessels and the volume of blood throughout your brain. The better the blood circulation in your brain, the better nourished your brain cells will be, resulting in higher cognitive performance, learning ability, and recall.

In addition, exercise improves neuroplasticity, or the capacity of the brain to change and cultivate new connections between neurons. Neuroplasticity is critical to integrating new brain cells into existing neural networks, allowing them to function properly and thus facilitating learning and memory. Scientists are not exactly sure *how* exercise encourages neuroplasticity, although one known effect is that exercise boosts the body's production of two chemicals called insulin growth factor (IGF-1) and brain-derived neurotrophic factor (BDNF), both of which stimulate the growth of new brain cells and support the maintenance of existing neural networks. Essentially, exercise can help your brain rewire itself, creating fresh associations and strengthening old ones.

Finally, exercise seems to boost various neurotransmitter systems in the brain, increasing circulating levels of dopamine, serotonin, GABA, and acetylcholine. This has a number of effects. Perhaps most famously, these higher volumes of dopamine and serotonin, your "pleasure" neurotransmitters, make exercise a great natural way to treat depression and other mood disorders. But more generally, high levels of neurotransmitters are also critical to improving cognition and memory, in part because they seem to help stimulate the production of BDNF and IGF.

Regardless of how exercise stimulates and sustains your brain, the results are clear and unequivocal. Spatial memory (your ability to remember where things are placed), semantic memory (your ability to remember words and facts), and executive function (the ability to plan and execute tasks) are all significantly improved. In addition, exercise increases the ability to both consolidate (create) and retrieve memories; it also enhances learning more generally.

Physical activity significantly improves brain function and cognition in people of all ages and fitness levels, and may in fact be particularly useful in older populations for its ability to prevent or slow brain deterioration. By working a regular exercise regimen into your week, you will be able to think and recall better and more quickly than you might ordinarily.

HOW MUCH EXERCISE SHOULD YOU GET?

Currently, both the CDC and the ACSM recommend that adults get about two and a half hours (150 minutes) of moderate-intensity aerobic activity each week. Moderate-intensity aerobic activity is defined as movement that raises your heart rate and makes you break a sweat. An easy way to tell whether your exertion level is moderate is that you'll be able to talk, but not sing, while performing the activity. Examples include a brisk walk, water aerobics, a leisurely bike ride, doubles tennis, ballroom danc-ing, or household activities like pushing a lawn mower or raking leaves. To meet your requirements, you could simply go for a half-hour stroll five times a week.

Alternatively, you can increase the intensity of your aerobic workout and decrease the amount of time you spend performing it. If you'd pre-fer this, the CDC recommends an hour and fifteen minutes (75 minutes) of vigorous-intensity aerobic activity, which is defined as movement that makes you breathe hard and fast, and causes your heart rate to increase significantly. Unlike moderate-intensity activity, vigorous exercise will make it very difficult to say more than a few words at a time without stopping to take a breath. Examples include running or jogging, swim-ming laps, playing singles tennis, jumping rope, and performing heavy-duty yardwork such as digging a new garden bed.

And, of course, you can mix up the times and intensities of your workouts. The rule of thumb is that one minute of vigorous-intensity activity equals two minutes of moderate-intensity activity. However you get it, your total should add up to about 150 minutes of moderate-intensity activity each week for basic results. So, for example, on Monday you could take a twenty-minute walk through the park, on Wednesday you could spend half an hour vacuuming the house, and on Friday you could take a fifty-minute indoor cycling class at your local gym. Because this last activity is fairly high in intensity, its minutes count twice—bringing your total up to the recommended 150 minutes of moderate activity.

In addition to your aerobic workout, the CDC and ACSM recom-mend that you also try to work in muscle-strengthening activities (anaer-obic activity) at least two times a week. Whether you meet these guidelines through weightlifting, resistance training, yoga, or gardening, this muscle-strengthening activity should engage all your major muscle groups (legs, hips, back, abdomen, chest, shoulders, and arms) for best results. While researchers consider the cognitive benefits of strength training to be generally less dramatic than that of aerobic exercise, there is evidence that muscle-building activities may actually impact areas of the brain that are untouched by a cardio workout. Moreover, studies show that any kind of physical activity, be it aerobic or nonaerobic, is bet-ter than none, at least where your memory is concerned.

If you haven't exercised for a while, consider the following tips. Start slowly, building up toward a longer workout period over time. Do not overexert yourself—excessive exercise can hurt your body and lead to inflammation. Make sure you warm up first by stretching. Even with mild exercise you may discover that you wake up sore the next day; however, you'll quickly see that the rewards of maintaining a weekly exercise regimen greatly outweigh your aches and pains. Work out with a partner; this helps keep both of you focused on your routine. And find a gym nearby—the easier and more convenient it is to get there, the more frequently you'll go.

If you have a heart condition, or if you are over the age of forty and have not been engaging in physical activity on a regular basis, you may want to consult with your healthcare provider before beginning a serious exercise program. Your doctor may perform a physical examination and possibly a stress test in order to ensure that your body can withstand sustained exertion.

CONCLUSION

It is important to understand that regular physical activity—no matter how vigorous—is not enough to offset a sedentary lifestyle. For best results, you must endeavor to be more active in all aspects of your daily routine. If you have a job that requires you sit at a desk for long periods of time, try to get up and move or stretch a little every hour. If you like to watch television, lift weights or do sit-ups during the commercial breaks. When your sister phones to update you on her latest achievement, take the call outside and go for a walk while chatting. And, when given the option, use the stairs, not the elevator.

The benefits for both your body and your mind will be enormous. As you have seen, any form of physical activity can actually grow your brain and improve blood circulation and neurotransmission within it. These changes have the effect of significantly enhancing cognition and memory. So get up off of the couch and start moving today!

9

Mental Activity

Use it or lose it—that's what many doctors and scientists say about your brain. While physical exercise is essential for improving your ability to think and remember, mental exercise is also very important. Just as you'd keep a vintage car up and running by taking it out for a spin on a regular basis, you need to keep your mind active in order to ensure good working condition. Medical studies have shown that cognitive stimulation—talking about the news with a friend, doing crosswords, playing music, or making art—can help you maintain your memory and potentially prevent against dementia. Social stimulation can be equally significant: by maintaining or developing your network of friends, relatives, and acquaintances, you can also help preserve and even improve your brain power.

Scientists don't yet understand exactly how cognitive and social activity affect the brain. Some believe that mental activity enhances neuroplasticity, or the brain's capacity to change and cultivate new connections between neurons. Others believe that a lifetime of consistent intellectual and social stimulation can lead to better *cognitive reserve*, or the capacity of the brain to tolerate age-related changes and damage. In one long-term, large-scale study of 13,000 elderly Britons, an active cognitive lifestyle was associated with less cerebrovascular disease (disease of the blood vessels in the brain), greater brain weight, and greater neuronal density and thickness of the frontal lobe. Following 2,802 Americans with normal cognitive and functional status, the 2006 Advanced Cognitive Training for Independent and Vital Elderly (ACTIVE) Study found that those who were taught strategies for remembering word lists and sequences saw both short- and long-term improvement in their overall memory and cognitive function.

Because the effects of cognitive and social exercise can be difficult to quantify over time, there have been relatively few other reliable studies conducted on the subject. Generally, however, scientists and doctors almost unanimously champion the benefits of exercising your brain. This chapter provides an overview of techniques and activities that invigorate your brain and thus boost your memory and general cognition. Whether you are forty, fifty, sixty, or older, by engaging your mind consistently and in a variety of ways, you will be able to stay sharp and focused for years to come.

MENTAL STAGNATION

For many people who have devoted their lifetimes to their jobs, there comes a time when they can no longer work at their positions. It may be an individual choice, or it may be a choice dictated by company policy. Some people have relationships and engagements outside of the office; they know that retirement does not mean retiring from an active life. Others wake up one morning and have no idea what to do with themselves. While some do find new purpose, too many retirees wind up withdrawing socially, biding their time and doing very little in the manner of physical or mental activity. The signs are very obvious. In general, they:

- Become socially inactive

- Watch a lot of television

- Use services that relieve them of their daily responsibilities

- Limit their travel

- Seek comfort and avoid challenging themselves in any way

In short, they have resigned themselves to watching the days go by. Perhaps you know a few people who fit this description. Odds are good that their lack of mental activity will most likely result in some form of memory loss. But it certainly doesn't have to be that way. As you will see, by stimulating the brain appropriately, metal stagnation does not have to happen to you.

MENTAL ENRICHMENT

As you have seen, it is vitally important to challenge your brain in order to keep it active and healthy. Mental exercise can lessen and improve normal age-related memory loss and mild cognitive impairment; although it cannot prevent dementia, consistent cognitive stimulation can potentially delay its onset. The following is a list of some things you can do to stimulate your mind.

- **Read a book.** While reading is generally a great way to work your brain, for extra challenge, try reading a book on a subject you wouldn't normally select. If you prefer mystery novels, pick up a book on economics or home cooking; if your reading is usually limited to the newspaper, try a book of short stories or other fiction.

- **Do crossword puzzles or other word games**. This helps maintain your semantic memory.

- **Memorize phone numbers, grocery lists, or other tidbits of information**. While a post-it note or a smartphone can easily store this information for you, by forcing your brain to remember a small piece of information, you can help exercise your memory. Or try memorizing a poem—any little thing can help.

- **Take music lessons**. Studies consistently show that musical training can bolster verbal ability and other types of cognition.

- **Learn a new language**. Being able to speak and distinguish between two or more languages can increase cognitive reserve. One study indicates that bilingual patients with Alzheimer's disease showed significantly less brain atrophy than monolingual patients.

- **Enroll in a class at your local college or community center**. By learning a new skill or acquiring new information, you encourage brain activity.

- **Do calculations in your head**. Instead of using a calculator or computer, try to do simple math problems by yourself.

- **Make art**. Exercise your creative side by painting, sculpting, or drawing.

- **Get lost**. Travel to an unfamiliar place—another state or even just a part of town you rarely visit. Ditch your GPS and try to navigate your way around the area using a map or even just your sense of space or direction.

- **Learn to play**. As an adult, the act of playing shapes the brain, opens the imagination, and enables you to be innovative and problem-solve.

With any mental activity, the key is always to take yourself out of your comfort zone. As Dr. Anne Fabiny, chief of geriatrics at the Cambridge Health Alliance says, "If it's too easy, it's not helping you." The harder you push yourself, the better the results for your brain. Make sure to engage in active learning—while it can be helpful to simply watch a lecture or a musical performance, the best mental exercises are those that force you to participate. Most important, try to challenge yourself on a regular basis throughout your life. Studies show that people who make a habit of learning new things reap the greatest and most enduring cognitive benefits.

SOCIAL STIMULATION

A diverse and well-developed social network is just as important as intellectual stimulation when it comes to keeping your mind nimble. Studies consistently show that people who are socially isolated or who have a limited or poor-quality network of friends and family are at a greater risk for memory loss and cognitive decline. An active social environment can also potentially help protect against various forms of dementia, including Alzheimer's disease. The following is a list of ways that you can cultivate a rich and rewarding social life:

- **Make regular dates with friends and family**. Protect against isolation by scheduling running engagements—Saturday morning coffee with your best friend, a weekly game of golf with your coworker, or Sunday dinner with your extended family. By creating a routine of social interaction, you can make sure you never lack for company or interpersonal stimulation.

- **Join a group**. Find like-minded individuals by joining a group that specializes in an activity you enjoy—sing in a choir, play in a community orchestra, join a local card group or book club.

- **Take a class**. Not only do classes offer ample mental stimulation, they sponsor conversation and provide opportunities to meet new people.

- **Get a job**. If you are capable and interested, try undertaking a new job. Even the smallest job affords opportunities for both mental and social activity; in addition, it can also give you a sense of purpose and a side income.

- **Start a business**. Have you ever considered turning a serious hobby into a professional pursuit? Self-employment offers many challenges and many rewards.

- **Play team sports**. Join a local soccer league or tennis tournament to meet new people and get fit at the same time.

- **Play a strategy game**. Games like chess, bridge, or mahjong require social interaction, and exercise your executive function and memory as well, encouraging you to plan several steps ahead of the immediate goal. While it's great to get involved in a league or club that gets you out of the house, many games are also available online, and can promote equally satisfying social interaction.

- **Play trivia**. Throughout North America, many bars and restaurants offer trivia nights. Some are even associated with national trivia organizations that allow you to compete against either the local establishment or players around the country. A little competition is healthy, and exercises both your social and mental skills.

- **Take up dancing**. Like team sports, dancing is a great way to spend time with others while also reaping the benefits of physical activity.

- **Get involved**. Community service and volunteer work allow you to do good while fostering friendships and relationships. Build new homes, work at a soup kitchen, or read to a small child.

- **Volunteer as a docent**. Thousands of organizations—museums, parks, town tourism bureaus, and libraries—are looking for people to become docents, or educational guides. As a docent, you will both learn and teach new information, all while meeting people and helping out your community.

- **Stay in touch**. If you have friends or family who don't live within traveling distance, keep up your connections by calling, writing, or emailing.

While it's important to simply get out of the house and spend time with new people, you don't need to become the life of the party in order to develop a healthy and valuable social network. In fact, some studies show that it's not the quantity of your social connections that matters, but rather the quality. In other words, two or three deep and meaningful relationships can sometimes be more invigorating than twenty more superficial friendships. Pursue the friendships that mean the most to you; quality relationships should provide support, comfort, and stimulation.

The advantages of taking part in group activities don't end with social enrichment. Many of the above activities offer additional benefits in the forms of physical or mental exercise. By participating in these multifaceted pastimes, you can thus stimulate different areas of your brain in different ways, providing broader support for your cognition and memory.

CONCLUSION

Many of the activities recommended above are absolutely free and allow you to get involved easily. The object for all of these activities is to keep your mind in peak condition. As you have seen, both mental and social stimulation are integral to maintaining and even improving your cognitive function as you age. Moreover, studies show that mental exercise and an active social network can help protect against other health problems, including cardiovascular disease—and even contribute to a longer life overall! For better memory and focus, get out there and challenge yourself. Your brain will thank you.

10

Sleep

Getting a good night's sleep is very important when it comes to maintaining good memory and focus. During sleep, your brain recharges, restoring the levels of hormones and neurotransmitters that support mental acuity and building new connections between neurons. As we discussed in Chapter 6, lack of sleep can significantly impair your ability to learn and recall information. In addition, prolonged sleep loss can set the stage for a number of other health conditions that also impact your cognitive function, including cardiovascular disease, weight gain, depression, and hormone and neurotransmitter imbalances.

That said, losing as little as one hour of sleep each night can have immediate consequences for your cognitive ability. How you sleep at night has a direct effect on how you feel and function the next day. Your brain needs at least six and a half hours of sleep each night in order to perform properly; any less than that and you will find yourself struggling to remember details, learn new information, or execute even the most straightforward mental tasks. Short-term sleep loss can also lower your mood, making you feel overly sensitive, emotional, or depressed. Accordingly, in order to maintain or enhance your memory and focus, it is important that you do optimize both the quality and quantity of your sleep.

While there are many treatment options available to people who suffer from chronic, or long-term insomnia (see Chapter 6), there are also a number of simple tips and techniques that can significantly help anybody who wants to get more restorative sleep. In addition, there is a variety of dietary supplements that you can take in order to remedy or prevent sleep loss. This chapter provides a basic overview of proper sleep habits and other easy ways to improve your sleep. For better sleep—and better memory—read on!

LIFESTYLE CHANGES

By making a few changes to the practices and habits that surround your normal sleep routine, you may be able to reduce, cure, or even prevent short-term or acute insomnia. Even if you don't suffer from sleep loss on a regular basis, the following tips can help you get the most out of your nights—so that you can get the most out of your days.

Avoid Alcohol Before Bedtime

While alcohol generally acts as a sedative, and thus may be a tempting solution to those who have trouble getting to sleep, studies show that alcohol consumed within six hours of bedtime can actually disrupt the second half of the sleep cycle, leading to restless or partial sleep. For some, alcohol can even worsen existing insomnia or sleep deprivation. For this reason, avoid drinking alcohol within six hours of the time you usually go to bed.

Avoid Aspartame

This artificial sweetener has been linked to higher risk of insomnia.

Avoid Caffeine Before Bedtime

Caffeine is a stimulant, and can keep you awake when you'd rather be sleeping. Although some people are less sensitive to caffeine than others, it's generally best to avoid consuming caffeinated products (coffee, tea, chocolate, some sodas) within six hours of the time you usually go to bed.

Don't Watch the Clock

There's nothing worse than lying in bed and watching the minutes tick by on your bedside clock. This behavior only adds to your stress and anxiety, making it harder to sleep. Avoid looking at your clock, or, better yet—keep clocks out of the bedroom entirely.

Eat Five to Six Small Meals A Day

For some, low blood sugar in the middle of the night can stimulate the production of hormones that wake you up, including epinephrine, glucagon, cortisol, and growth hormone. To regulate your blood sugar, eat five to six smaller meals throughout the day instead of the traditional three larger ones. A small snack before bedtime can actually help you stay asleep: a banana is a good choice because it contains both magnesium and tryptophan, two substances that promote better rest (see pages 138 to 139).

Establish a Bedtime Routine

Try to create a routine that you follow every evening in the half hour or so before you go to bed, like reading a book in another room, drinking some warm milk, listening to soothing music, or taking a hot shower. After a while, these rituals will start to cue your body into the idea that it's time to go to bed.

Exercise Regularly

Research shows that regular exercise can promote sleep and prevent the development of chronic insomnia. Exercise decreases stress and boosts your serotonin levels (see page 102), making it easier for you to fall asleep. It is best to exercise either in the morning or in the early afternoon; exercise shortly before bed can invigorate you and keep you awake.

Get Plenty of Sunlight During the Day

Sunlight helps maintain your circadian rhythms, including your sleep-wake cycle.

Go To Bed When You're Actually Tired

It's important to be able to recognize when your body is physically ready to go to bed, and when you're merely fatigued mentally.

Improve Your Sleeping Environment

Studies show that a dark, cool, quiet bedroom is the best possible environment for sleep. Make sure to cover your windows with shades, blinds, or curtains—sunlight can jumpstart your sleep-wake cycle, causing you to rise earlier than you'd prefer. If you live in a city or another location where noise is an issue, consider investing in earplugs or a white noise machine to help you block out any sounds that might wake you or keep you from sleeping.

Keep Pets Out of the Bedroom

It may be difficult to say no to Cleo or Fido, but your pets can sometimes interfere with a proper night's rest. Pets operate on a different sleep-wake cycle than we do, and unless you want to be harnessed to their idea of when to rise, it's best to keep them out of the bedroom.

Maintain a Fixed Sleep Schedule

For better sleep, it's important that you maintain a stable routine, with set bedtimes and wake-up times. Decide what time you want to go to bed and what time you want to wake up—and stick to those hours every day! Changing your schedule from day to day disrupts your circadian rhythms (see page 93), and can result in poor or reduced sleep.

Manage Pain

If muscle, joint, or nerve pain is keeping you up at night, make sure you take a pain reliever right before bedtime. It's important that the effects of the medication last through the night, so that you don't wake up in pain and then have trouble getting back to sleep.

No Napping!

Avoid taking naps during the day, as these can prevent you from getting a full night's sleep later.

Use Breathing Exercises and Other Relaxation Techniques to Fall Asleep

If you are anxious or tense because of stress, techniques like progressive muscle relaxation, prayer, meditation, and breathing exercises can help you fall asleep more quickly.

Use Your Bed for Sleep and Sex Only

Behavioral therapists believe that by strengthening the association between your bed and sleep, you will be able to fall asleep faster. Don't read, watch television, or use your laptop or tablet while you are in bed.

By limiting your time in the bedroom to the hours you sleep or have sex, you mentally establish that the bedroom is a place for these two activities only. If you can't get to sleep within half an hour of lying down, get up and move to another room, so as not to destabilize the association.

STRESS MANAGEMENT

Stress is a major cause of acute or short-term insomnia. If you're under a lot of stress—say you've got a big deadline coming up at work, or you've had a fight with your spouse—you may not be able to sleep properly. This is because stress makes your body produce more cortisol, a hormone that plays a major role in regulating your sleep-wake cycle.

Under normal circumstances, your body's natural cortisol concentration peaks in the early morning, telling your body to wake up. From that point on, your cortisol level declines, reaching its lowest point about an hour before you normally go to sleep, when, deprived of this "go" hormone, you finally nod off. About two hours after midnight, your body once more begins to produce cortisol, gradually increasing production until the level peaks and you wake again. When this cycle progresses the way nature intended, your waking hours are productive and your sleep is deep and restful.

Unfortunately, the normal ebb and flow of cortisol is easily disrupted by stress. Stress forces your body to produce more cortisol on a regular basis in order to deal with the pressures of daily life. With higher levels of this "wake-up" hormone in your system—particularly at night, when cortisol levels should be at their lowest—many people find it hard to go to sleep. Sometimes stress can even cause the cortisol cycle of production to reverse itself, with your cortisol level peaking during normal sleeping time and reaching its lowest point upon awakening. As a result, you're anxious and alert when you should be sleeping, and groggy and tired when you should be energized.

Because stress thus interferes with your sleep cycle, it's important to take steps to control it. While you won't be able to eliminate all sources of stress from your life, you can certainly reduce their effects by using any of the stress management strategies discussed in Chapter 11. By following these guidelines, you may find that you are able to significantly cut down on your stress—and thus limit its impact on your sleep and memory!

DIETARY SUPPLEMENTS

In addition to improving your sleep habits and managing your stress, you can also take certain vitamins, minerals, amino acids, and botanicals that will help relieve or even prevent sleep loss.

Supplement	Dosage	Considerations
California Poppy (*Eschscholzia californica*)	Use as directed.	Extract concentrations vary from brand to brand; for this reason, it is best to follow dosage instructions as indicated on label.
Chamomile	Drink as a tea three to four times daily.	Do not use in conjunction with other sedatives, including alcohol. Should not be taken with anticoagulants or by anyone whose blood does not clot easily.
5-hydroxytryp-tophan (5-HTP)	50 to 300 mg daily.	Can be taken with magnesium for increased effectiveness. May interfere with antidepressants. Should not be taken with medications for Parkinson's disease. Consult with your doctor before taking if you have diabetes, high blood pressure, heart disease, or an autoimmune disorder.
Hops	Use as directed.	Extract concentrations vary from brand to brand; for this reason, it is best to follow dosage instructions as indicated on label.
Lavender	Use as directed.	Extract concentrations vary from brand to brand; for this reason, it is best to follow dosage instructions as indicated on label.
Lemon balm	Use as directed.	Do not take if you have glaucoma.
L-theanine	100 to 200 mg, taken in the morning and evening.	Extract concentrations vary from brand to brand; for this reason, it is best to follow dosage instructions as indicated on label.
Magnesium	400 to 600 mg daily.	May cause loose stools.
Magnolia officinalis	Use as directed.	Extract concentrations vary from brand to brand; for this reason, it is best to follow dosage instructions as indicated on label.
Melatonin	0.5 to 3 mg daily.	High doses may cause dizziness, headaches, insomnia, or depression. May amplify the effects of medications that lower blood pressure, or increase blood sugar levels in some diabetics.
Passionflower	Use as directed.	High doses may cause irregular heartbeat (arrhythmia). May interfere with monoamine oxidase (MAO) inhibitors.

Supplement	Dosage	Considerations
Tryptophan	2,000 mg daily.	Avoid protein intake just before use. Can be taken with vitamin B_6, B_3, or magnesium for maximum effectiveness. May interfere with selective serotonin reuptake inhibitors (SSRIs) or monoamine oxidase (MAO) inhibitors.
Valerian (*Valeriana officinalis*)	Use as directed.	Should be taken with vitamin B_6, B_3, or magnesium for maximum effectiveness. Can cause headaches, dizziness, restlessness, heart palpitations, or gastrointestinal disturbances. Should not be taken by women who are pregnant or nursing.
Vitamin B_1 (thiamine)	10 to 100 mg daily.	High doses may deplete your body of vitamin B_6 (pyridoxine) and magnesium.
Vitamin B_3 (niacinamide)	50 to 3,000 mg daily.	Sedative effects may be amplified by simultaneously taking L-tryptophan. Can cause skin flushing, sensations of heat, stomach problems, or dry skin. Consult with your doctor if taking more than 100 mg daily; higher doses can cause liver damage, peptic ulcers, or glucose intolerance. Should not be taken by those who suffer from liver disease, or at the same time as other B-complex vitamins.
Vitamin B_{12} (cobalamin)	800 to 1,000 mcg daily.	May cause diarrhea, blood clots, itching, or allergic reactions. Consult with your healthcare provider before using if you have high blood pressure or other forms of heart disease.
Ziziphus spinosa	Use as directed.	Extract concentrations vary from brand to brand; for this reason, it is best to follow dosage instructions as indicated on label.

CONCLUSION

As you have read, a full night's rest is essential to maintaining your memory and focus. If you suspect you are not getting enough sleep, or that the sleep you are getting is of poor quality, there are many steps you can take to remedy this underlying problem. The techniques, strategies, and supplements discussed in this chapter will help optimize your ability to fall asleep and stay asleep. Get better sleep—and see immediate improvements in your focus and recall!

11

Stress Management

All of us experience stress to some degree or another on a daily basis. When we do, our bodies automatically release special hormones in order to manage the tough situations we find ourselves in. The release of stress hormones is part of a basic survival mechanism that allowed our ancient ancestors to react quickly in order to protect themselves from a perceived threat. Confronted with danger (such as the approach of a sabre-toothed tiger), these hormones furnished our ancestors with a temporary burst of energy and enhanced cardiac and musculoskeletal performance, so that they could either combat the threat or escape it. Accordingly, this biochemical reaction is known as the "fight-or-flight" response. Once the danger passed, the hormones dissipated and life went on as before.

The "fight-or-flight" response is a built-in part of our bodies' evolutionary design, triggered not just by acute or short-term episodes of perceived danger, but by any situation we interpret as stressful. Whether you are being chased by a sabre-toothed tiger or facing a looming deadline at work, your body's response is the same: stress hormones are released to help you cope. The trouble is, for so many of us today, stress is no longer an acute (temporary) reaction to an immediate threat. As we deal with work-related pressure, relationship issues, and financial worries, stress is increasingly experienced as a chronic, long-term reaction, with stress hormones continually released in an ongoing and seemingly futile attempt to clear the stubborn source of the problem.

This chronic stress response can have a devastating impact on your body—and your mind. As you saw in Chapter 4, stress can wreak havoc on your brain. Excess levels of cortisol, your main stress hormone, can damage neurons and rewire existing electrical connections between them, leading to loss of brain function, particularly in the hippocampus (your memory center) and the amygdala (your emotional center). In effect, stress can seriously impair your memory and focus.

Not only does stress affect your mind directly—it also indirectly influences cognition by contributing to various conditions that independently impact your recall and mental acuity. As you will remember from Chapters 6 and 10, stress can contribute to sleep loss and insomnia; it can also raise your risk of heart disease, as seen in Chapter 2. In addition, high levels of cortisol can affect your other hormone and neurotransmitter levels, altering the chemical balance that is so integral to your brain's health.

Because stress is thus harmful to your mental acuity in many different ways, it is very important that you learn to control its impact on your life. This chapter provides you with a series of tips that will help protect you against the damaging influence of chronic stress. While you won't be able to eliminate all sources of stress from your life, you can certainly reduce their effects by using a number of the simple strategies outlined here. The less stressed you are, the sharper your mind will be for years to come.

IDENTIFY YOUR STRESSORS

Some sources of stress are acute and unpredictable—a flat tire, an untimely illness, or a late train—you have no way of knowing when these problems will pop up, though they usually resolve themselves quickly. But many more stressors are predictable, as they constitute long-term or chronic sources of frustration. It may seem obvious, but it is very important to be able to recognize the people, events, or situations that make you anxious, unhappy, or angry. What (or who) are your triggers? Sometimes your triggers will be clear—a pending business deal, a fight with your significant other, or a credit card bill that you can't pay. But sometimes stressors are less obvious: simply being busy, having too many commitments, or even making a big change to your life can make you feel overwhelmed and unable to cope. Take stock: what's working in your life right now? What isn't working? In order to successfully manage your problems, you must first identify them. Consider the most common sources of chronic stress:

- Work-related issues
- Personal relationships
- Family disputes and obligations
- Health issues
- Financial problems
- Environment (noise, toxins, etc.)

ELIMINATE AVOIDABLE STRESSORS

Many sources of chronic stress simply aren't going to disappear on their own; others, like financial difficulties or a rough patch in a relationship, may take time to resolve. But some stressors can in fact be removed. For example, if you like playing tennis, but hate having to participate in your club's competitive ladder, consider playing elsewhere—there's no reason to turn a fun activity into an onerous responsibility and source of stress. Sometimes stress comes from the feeling that you lack control; making the choice to remove yourself from a stressful situation can sometimes do a lot to restore that sense of control and improve your general outlook. This is not to say that you should eliminate all stressors from your life; a certain amount of change and challenge can be positive. And despite how crazy your children make you at times, for example, there are still many compelling reasons why you should probably keep them around. But if the cons outweigh the pros—if your stress becomes distress—it may be time to reconsider whether you really need a certain person or situation in your life.

REDUCE THE FREQUENCY OR INTENSITY OF YOUR STRESSORS

Because you won't always be able to eliminate all the sources of stress from your life, it's critical that you do what you can to loosen their grip on you. Try to reduce the frequency with which you have to deal with sources of stress, or dial down the intensity. If spending time with your parent makes you feel like tearing your hair out, see them less often, or find a fun, low-impact activity in which you can all participate without getting into an argument. If you've reached an impasse in a business negotiation, take a break. This can defuse the tension, allowing you to regain your perspective and calm; sometimes a little breathing room is all that's needed to make a stressful situation less acute.

TAKE CONTROL OF YOUR TIME

One of the most important things you can do to reduce your stress is to gain control over your time. Keep yourself busy, but don't overcommit. Figure out how much work and responsibility you can take on without feeling overwhelmed, and make sure to schedule time for yourself, for your family, and for your friends. As the poet Carl Sandburg once wrote, "Time is the coin of your life. It is the only coin you have, and only you can determine how it will be spent. Be careful lest you let other people spend it for you."

EXERCISE REGULARLY

Exercise is one of the best ways to combat stress. Exercise is not only good for your overall health; it also boosts production of certain neuro-transmitters that make you feel better and help promote sleep (see page 94). For best results, health experts recommend at least thirty minutes daily of moderate aerobic exercise, but any form of physical activity is better than none. More information on the benefits of exercise can be found in Chapter 8.

FIND AN OUTLET FOR YOUR ENERGIES

Stress can make you feel unusually alert or antsy, distracting you and making it difficult to concentrate. Put that nervous energy to work by taking up a fun activity: play a sport, go dancing, sing in a choir, acquire a hobby, or do some community service. By keeping yourself active and engaged, you'll be able to focus better and remember faster; you'll also sleep better at night. And, as you saw in Chapter 9, mental and social stimulation can be beneficial more generally when it comes to maintaining your mood and cognitive function. Alternatively, do something useful: clean out the attic, wash your car, or finish organizing that photo album. The completion of practical tasks can give you a sense of personal satisfaction, and remind you that with a little work, most obstacles can be overcome.

KEEP UP WITH FRIENDS AND FAMILY

It's important to have a strong support network, especially during stress-ful times. Spending time with people who care about you can help provide perspective on your situation, as well as emotional relief. Remember, it's the quality of your relationships that matters, not the number. A meaningful interaction with a friend or family member can bring you food for thought and peace of mind.

LEARN TO RELAX

You can train your body and mind to relax by taking part in tai chi, yoga, or other meditative practices. Many of us actually hold their breath or forget to breathe normally when we're stressed out; breathing exercises can help control immediate reactions to stress and also ease transitions into sleep at night. Look for a yoga class that is conveniently located near you.

LET YOUR FEELINGS OUT

Don't bottle up your anxieties—you'll only make them worse. Instead, express yourself; learn to identify the sources of your stress so that you are better able to deal with them. If you don't feel comfortable talking about your problems with a friend or family member, consider consulting with a therapist or religious advisor. And in case you find face-to-face discussions stressful, there are many helpful websites with chat rooms that you can use.

EAT A WHOLESOME, WELL-BALANCED DIET

As discussed in Chapter 12, a wholesome, well-balanced diet can make a big difference to your overall health and wellbeing. By making sure your body has all the nutrients it needs, you can help protect against certain physiological or environmental sources of stress. In addition, you should be aware that chronic stress can deplete your body of many essential nutrients, including magnesium, potassium, B vitamins, vitamin C, zinc, and taurine. Accordingly, you may wish to supplement your diet in order to make sure that you have adequate supplies of these vital substances.

AVOID TOXINS

Similarly, avoid toxins—chemicals that act as poisons in your body. Toxins are essentially environmental stressors that can damage your body and prevent your mind from functioning properly. In addition to the heavy metals discussed in Chapter 3, you may want to consider reducing or eliminating your exposure to sugar and sugar substitutes, caffeine, nicotine, alcohol, and drugs; these chemicals can be very harmful to your brain and body. If you have any food allergies or intolerances, avoid contact with these substances.

TAP INTO YOUR SPIRITUALITY

Some studies show that belief in a higher power can help you deal with stress by providing perspective and comfort. Let your faith help you carry your burdens. Consider attending a religious service or talking with a spiritual counselor. Remember, there are a number of nondenominational groups that can provide strong spiritual support as well.

BE POSITIVE

Sometimes we can be our own worst enemies; negativity or cynicism can easily get in the way of a healthy, productive life. Studies have shown that optimists tend to have increased lifespans, more responsive immune systems, and lower risk of cardiovascular disease. They also cope with stress better. So try to keep your outlook positive and eliminate what therapists call negative "self-talk," the interior monologue that you have with yourself. Don't put yourself down, and remind yourself that everything will most likely turn out fine in the long run. If you're trying to meet a deadline at work, don't tell yourself you'll never get it done or that your boss won't like the results. Remind yourself that your boss hired you for good reasons, and that you've gotten your work in on time before. Most obstacles can be overcome; if you can remember that, all challenges will be more easily managed.

CONCLUSION

Stress can take over your life—if you let it. If you are reading this chapter, however, chances are good that you've already made a commitment toward a calmer, more mindful life. This commitment is the first step toward lowering your stress. By following the guidelines above, you will be able to significantly cut down on your stress, and thus limit its impact on your memory and cognitive function!

12

Diet

When it comes to supporting your mind, one of the most important things you can do is to adopt a healthy, well-balanced diet. As you have seen throughout this book, the substances you put into your body can have a profound effect on your cognitive function and memory. Nowhere is this more true than where your diet is concerned. Based around processed foods, sugars, simple carbohydrates, and saturated and trans fats, the standard American diet is responsible for many of the serious health problems that plague our country today. Most important, the standard American diet does no favors for your brain. It contributes to weight gain, heart disease, chronic inflammation, and hormonal imbalance—all conditions that can impair your mental acuity, as you have read.

Clearly, a change in American eating habits is in order. For decades, scientists all over the world have championed the Mediterranean diet as the safest and most effective nutritional regimen for encouraging better overall health and longevity. Drawing from the culinary traditions of Crete, Greece, and Southern Italy, the Mediterranean diet emphasizes fruits, vegetables, fish, legumes, and whole grains, and limits the consumption of red meat and unhealthy fats. For best results, doctors advise patients to also adopt the strong social ties and physically active lifestyle associated with the Mediterranean diet.

The results of the diet are well known. Beginning with the Seven Countries Study, a long-term and cross-cultural examination of heart attack risk initiated in the 1950s, countless reports and reviews have confirmed the diet's advantages in promoting cardiovascular health. In addition, subsequent research has linked the Mediterranean diet to lower rates of cancer, diabetes, and reduced mortality rates overall.

But the benefits of the Mediterranean diet are not limited to your body. Strikingly, recent studies have also indicated that a Mediterranean-style diet can be of enormous help to your brain, significantly slowing mental decline and even protecting against mild cognitive impairment and various forms of dementia, including Alzheimer's disease. One recent study estimated that high adherence to a Mediterranean diet was associated with 28 percent less risk of developing mild cognitive impairment and 40 percent less risk of developing Alzheimer's disease in older patients. Not only does the Mediterranean diet help control various risk factors—including cardiovascular disease and chronic inflammation—that contribute to the likelihood of dementia, but it also features various vitamins, antioxidants, and other nutrients that independently maintain and enhance brain function.

Because of the Mediterranean diet's many advantages, it has been recommended by many established health institutions, including the World Health Organization, the American Heart Association, and the Mayo and Cleveland Clinics. But adopting a Mediterranean-style diet is in no way a burden. One of the reasons that the Mediterranean diet is so successful is that despite the changes you may have to make, you still get to eat very tasty, satisfying food. Accordingly, this chapter offers some basic guidelines for adopting a Mediterranean-style eating plan. By feeding your body right, you can effectively nourish your mind!

AVOID SUGAR AND PROCESSED FOODS

Avoid sugar and sugar substitutes like aspartame. These substances can act as toxins, causing chronic inflammation and upsetting your hormonal balance (See Chapters 5 and 4). Instead, the Mediterranean diet encourages you to satisfy your sweet tooth with fruit (see right). Choose whole fruit, not fruit juices, as even unsweetened juices can contain as much sugar as a soda. If you really need to boost the sweetness of a certain dish, use a natural substance, like honey or agave nectar.

Similarly, avoid or eliminate processed foods from your diet. Studies suggest that new food processing techniques such as extreme heating, irradiation, ionization, pasteurization, and sterilization may promote low-grade chronic inflammation by contributing to glycation (abnormal cross-linking of proteins) and oxidation of proteins and lipids. Certain food preparations at home amount to processing, too: frying, broiling, and grilling your food can also increase glycation.

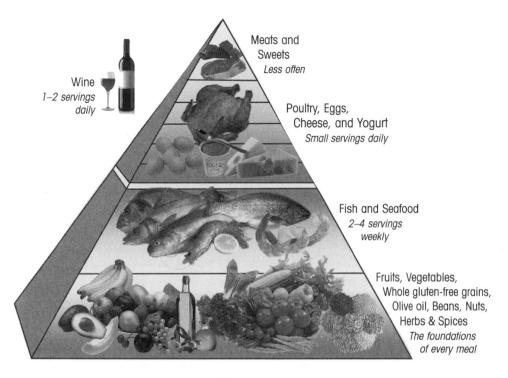

Figure 12.1. **The Mediterranean Diet Pyramid**

Instead of using these preparation methods, try lightly steaming, boiling, poaching, and stewing your food; this may help decrease the formation of these substances.

EAT LOTS OF FRUITS AND VEGETABLES

Plant foods are a central element of the Mediterranean diet. Besides tasting good, plant foods provide many significant benefits. For one thing, fruits and nonstarchy vegetables are low in calories but rich in nutrients that are integral to brain health, including vitamins A and C. Often, these nutrients come in the form of antioxidants—special vitamins and minerals that help fight against inflammation and free radical damage in your nervous system and elsewhere. Fruits and vegetables are also full of fiber—these indigestible carbohydrates make you feel full and help reduce the risk of heart disease and gastrointestinal disorders—and contain special compounds called plant sterols, which limit the amount of cholesterol absorbed by your digestive system.

Along with whole grains, fruits and vegetables should be the foundation on which every meal should be based. Aim to get between four to eight servings of nonstarchy vegetables and two to four servings of fruit each day. Traditionally, the Mediterranean diet makes extensive use of tomatoes, which contain the powerful antioxidant lycopene, itself linked to lower rates of certain types of cancer. One initial study shows that lycopene's use in reducing free radical damage and oxidative stress may also result in better cognitive function. For even more nutritional punch, doctors recommend that people eat plenty of leafy greens (spinach, Swiss chard) and cruciferous vegetables (*Brassica*) like broccoli and kale. These vegetables contain high levels of antioxidants and other phytochemicals that fight inflammation and cancer, and will help keep your body and mind healthy for years to come. You should also try to choose fruits that are full of fiber and antioxidants, like blueberries, blackberries, cherries, peaches, plums, and raspberries. To maximize the nutrient content of the plant foods you eat, pick those that are fresh, organic, seasonal, and locally grown.

EAT GLUTEN-FREE GRAINS

Although whole grains are traditionally essential to the Mediterranean diet, many of them contain a special type of protein called gluten. Today, a significant portion of the American population has either a sensitivity to gluten (a condition called gluten intolerance) or an allergy to it (a more serious disorder called celiac disease)—and research suggests that these numbers will only grow in the next century. Many people aren't even aware that they're allergic to gluten, and often, this condition is misdiagnosed as irritable bowel syndrome or another gastrointestinal disorder. By one estimate, there are thirty undiagnosed sufferers for every person diagnosed with celiac disease.

Due to the prevalence of gluten intolerances and allergies, I recommend limiting your consumption of grains that contain gluten, including wheat, rye, bulgur, couscous, semolina, barley and barley malt, triticale, einkorn, kamut, and American oatmeal. You don't need to cut out all cereals from your diet. Instead, try one of the following grains:

- Rice
- Wild rice
- Teff
- Corn
- Buckwheat
- Sorghum
- Millet
- Quinoa
- Amaranth

Unlike popular low-carbohydrate diets, the Mediterranean diet encourages you to eat ample portions of whole grains—four servings each day are recommended.

REPLACE "BAD" FATS WITH "GOOD" FATS

The Mediterranean diet is not a low-fat diet—by some estimates, calories derived from fat amount to about 30 percent of your entire intake. Rather, the Mediterranean diet distinguishes and chooses between the types of fats consumed. Instead of eating "bad" saturated and trans fats like butter, lard, and hydrogenated oils, the Mediterranean diet traditionally emphasizes the "good" unsaturated fat, olive oil, which is associated with lower rates of obesity, heart disease, and certain types of cancer. Olive oil also contains essential fats and antioxidants that can reduce inflammation and satisfy hunger for longer periods of time. More recently, medical professionals have also recommended the use of canola oil, which contains omega-3 and omega-6 fatty acids (see below).

INCORPORATE OMEGA-3 AND OMEGA-6 FATTY ACIDS INTO YOUR DIET

Omega fatty acids are essential fats, meaning that they are not made by your body, but are critical to your body's functioning, helping to maintain the integrity of your cells and facilitating nutrient transport. When consumed in appropriate amounts, omega fatty acids can fight inflammation, lower "bad" cholesterol, moderate blood pressure, and generally help reduce your risk of cardiovascular disease. Omega-3 fatty acids are found in pumpkin seeds, walnuts, dark leafy green vegetables, and cold-water fish, including salmon, halibut, and trout. Omega-6 fatty acids are found in many cold-pressed oils, including corn, canola, soy, sunflower, safflower, and sesame oils. Generally, dieticians recommend taking in omega-3 and omega-6 fatty acids in a balanced (one-to-one or two-to-one) ratio; some evidence indicates that an excess of omega-6 fatty acids can lead to inflammatory disorders such as rheumatoid arthritis and inflammatory bowel disease.

DRINK WINE—IN MODERATION!

The Mediterranean diet encourages limited consumption of alcohol. In fact, one study found that alcohol consumption was responsible for near-

ly 24 percent of the reduced mortality rate associated with the Mediterranean diet (high vegetable, fruit, and nut consumption accounted for a
combined 27 percent). Red wine is particularly recommended because it
contains many antioxidants, including a special chemical called resvera-
trol that seems to increase your "good" cholesterol, reduce the formation
of blood clots, and lower your risk for obesity, atherosclerosis (hardening
of the arteries), and heart disease more generally.

If you are going to drink, however, do so in moderation. Alcohol
can be addictive; drink too much and you can raise your blood pressure
and triglycerides, and increase your risk of liver disease and certain
types of cancer. Accordingly, doctors recommend that women limit
their intake to one drink a day (one beer, 4 oz of wine, or 1.5 oz of
80- or 100-proof spirits) and men limit theirs to two. If you are pregnant,
an alcoholic, or have liver damage or a weak heart, you should avoid
alcohol altogether.

EAT LESS RED MEAT AND MORE FISH, LEAN PROTEINS, AND NUTS

With its high levels of saturated fat, red meat is treated as a rare indul-
gence in the Mediterranean diet. Instead, your protein needs are satisfied
with fish from the ocean (especially those rich in omega fatty acids) and
poultry, which tends to be relatively lean and low in fat content. Doctors
generally recommend that you have one to three servings of poultry and
two servings of fish each week.

The Mediterranean diet also encourages you to eat more legumes—
beans, walnuts, pecans, almonds, sunflower seeds—which are high in
protein, fiber, iron, and many B vitamins. Nuts and seeds are rich in
unsaturated fat, which can increase your "good" cholesterol without
simultaneously raising the bad. Doctors recommend that you try to work
in about a handful of nuts eats day, and one to three servings of beans
and other legumes.

If you must have red meat from time to time, try eating lamb. Lamb
is high in omega-3 fatty acids and the amino acid carnitine. As you will
see in the next chapter, carnitine is an excellent nutrient that helps maintain your memory and focus.

Whenever possible, choose protein sources that are locally sourced
and organic. By eating organic, you can limit the volume of toxins that
enter your body, and help preserve the environment, as well.

Fish and Mercury

Traditionally, the Mediterranean diet relied heavily on fish as an excellent source of protein. While fish is generally considered to be a healthy choice, there are some precautions you should take before increasing your consumption dramatically. As you read in Chapter 3, most fish contain at least low levels of the heavy metal methyl mercury. Accordingly, doctors recommend paying attention to the types of fish you eat in order to limit your exposure to this toxic substance. Generally speaking, the bigger the fish, the greater its mercury content will likely be. In addition, certain farm-raised fish, like salmon, can have very high levels of mercury. Whenever possible, eat organic, wild, locally-sourced fish; these will have the highest nutrient levels and the lowest volume of toxins.

The following is an overview of the mercury content of fish commonly eaten in the United States:

Low Mercury Content (Safe to Eat Regularly): Wild salmon and organic farm-raised salmon, sardines, tilapia, orange roughy, catfish, shrimp, scallops, squid, oysters.

Moderate Mercury Content (Safe to Eat Occasionally): Ocean trout, flounder, mahi-mahi, red snapper, striped bass, cod, lobster, halibut.

High Mercury Content (Avoid or Eat Rarely): Chilean sea bass, shark, swordfish, grouper, tilefish, marlin, Spanish or king mackerel, bluefish, tuna.

LIMIT YOUR DAIRY INTAKE

Dairy products are not a large part of the Mediterranean diet, but they are a welcome addition—as long as they're low in fat content. Cheese and yogurt can be eaten in moderation, but milk consumption is traditionally low. If you really want to have a glass of milk, try a nonbovine source: goat milk, almond milk, and cashew milk are all great, healthy alternatives! Occasionally, you might also want to consider substituting omega-3-rich avocado for the cheese on your sandwich.

Generally, it is recommended that you have one to three servings of milk, yogurt, or cheese each day.

LIMIT OR AVOID SALTY FOODS

One of the many reasons that explain why the Mediterranean is so successful in lowering the risk of heart disease is that salty foods are limited or avoided altogether. High sodium (salt) intake is associated with high blood pressure and other cardiovascular problems; regardless of the specific diet cardiologists recommend, they almost always tell their patients to reduce their consumption of salt and salty foods. To compensate for any perceived loss of flavor, the Mediterranean diet advocates the use of spices and herbs to create new and exciting dishes. If you must eat a packaged or processed food now and then, try to avoid anything that has more than 500 mg of sodium per serving.

CONCLUSION

As you can see, the Mediterranean diet is not a diet of deprivation; it is a flexible and highly manageable way of life that encourages better health while still allowing for enjoyable, satisfying meals. While the best results will be attained by sticking closely to the guidelines listed above, studies show that even small changes to the way you eat—like swapping olive oil for butter or margarine—can make a big difference. The more faithfully you follow a Mediterranean-style diet, the better your results will be for both your body and your mind. So take care of your brain, and eat right!

13

Supplements

A s you saw in Chapter 12, a wholesome, well-balanced diet is critical to the good health of your brain and nervous system. Unfortunately, it is not always possible to get all the nutrients you need through diet alone. Modern agricultural practices have leached vital minerals from our cropland; as a result, the fruits and vegetables grown in that depleted soil simply do not contain plentiful nutrients. Moreover, the nutrients that remain begin to decline as soon as the plant food is picked. Cold storage continues the destruction of nutrient content. For example, stored grapes lose up to 30 percent of their B vitamins by the time they arrive in most grocery stores; stored asparagus can lose up to 90 percent of its vitamin C. Take fresh food home, and further nutrients are lost in the cooking process; eat prepared foods, and know that many nutrients have already been lost in the process of blanching, sterilizing, canning, milling, or freezing.

In an ideal world, we would be able to eat all our food within an hour of harvesting or slaughter, thus reaping their full benefits. Unfortunately, this simply isn't possible for the vast majority of us. Other factors also contribute to nutrient deficiencies: certain pharmaceutical drugs and even the aging process can prevent our bodies from making or using all the vitamins and minerals we need to function. As a result, we must look elsewhere to ensure that we get all the nutrients we need. This chapter will examine the vitamins, minerals, herbs, and other supplements that are most essential to supporting and enhancing your cognitive function. By adding these supplements to your daily routine, you can help protect your mind for years to come.

HOW TO USE SUPPLEMENTS

Clearly, it is important that you supplement your diet with certain nutrients in order to allow your mind to be the best that it can be. The problem
is, not all supplements are created equal—many different factors affect
the quality and absorption rates of the supplements you take. This section provides you with some basic information on how to choose and
take supplements for maximum effectiveness.

Choosing Supplements

There are four basic grades of dietary supplements, differing in terms of
quality. Supplements that are pharmaceutical grade meet the highest regulatory standards for purity, dissolution (ability to dissolve), and absorption. Pharmaceutical grade supplements are 99-percent pure, with no
added binders, fillers, dyes, or other unknown substances. Their quality
has been assured by an outside party—the United States Pharmacopeia
(USP). While pharmaceutical grade supplements can be harder to find
and are significantly more expensive than medical or nutritional grade
supplements, their high quality ensures the greatest benefits.

If you cannot buy pharmaceutical grade supplements, choose the
next-highest grade available to you—either medical or nutritional grade.
Because these lesser-grade supplements are less pure than pharmaceutical grade substances, they often contain lower volumes of the actual substance you're trying to consume. Accordingly, you may need to take
larger doses of these lesser-grade supplements in order to achieve the
desired effects. Here are some other considerations to keep in mind when
choosing a supplement:

- Check the ingredient list. Ideally, the supplement's ingredient list
  should have only one item on it: the nutrient itself. If that isn't possible, choose supplements that contain no preservatives or artificial col-
  oring. And, of course, make sure that the product contains no
  substances to which you may have an allergy or intolerance—soy,
  dairy, and gluten are sometimes used in supplement manufacturing.

- Choose supplements that are natural, not synthetic; natural forms tend
  to be more active and easily absorbed than synthetic versions.

- Many herbal supplements have been found to contain traces of heavy
  metals such as arsenic, lead, mercury, and cadmium. To avoid expos-

ing yourself to these toxins, look for herbs that carry seals of approval from regulatory agencies such as the USP, NSF International, or ConsumerLab.com. These groups help ensure that the product you consume has been tested and found free of contaminants.

- Each supplement should be packaged in a container that protects its contents from the light. Amber-colored glass is the best choice. Supplements should also be vacuum sealed to preserve freshness and ensure that nobody has tampered with the product. When you purchase a supplement, ask if it requires refrigeration.

Taking Supplements

The dosages of vitamins, minerals, and other nutritional supplements found throughout this book are designed for adults who have normal kidney and liver function. You will note that many dosages are greater than the dietary reference intakes (DRIs) recommended by the United States government. This is because the DRIs do not consider the amount of a nutrient needed to promote optimum health—they simply calculate the bare minimum needed to avoid nutritional deficiency. For best results, you'll need to take more than the DRIs suggest.

In some cases, I have recommended a dosage range instead of a specific amount. For example, on page 171, I suggest taking 60 to 120 milligrams of ginkgo. If you are working with a physician specializing in metabolic and anti-aging medicine, he or she will be able to determine the dosage within this range that is most appropriate for your specific medical status. If you are establishing a supplementation regimen on your own, however, I suggest that you start with the lowest possible dose and maintain it for two weeks. If you suffer no side effects but see no benefits in that time, you may want to increase the amount you are taking. If after two more weeks you still experience no improvement, increase the dose again, never exceeding the upper range of the dosage I have recommended. Not all supplements are effective for all people; if you have reached the maximum dosage of a supplement and still see no improvement, discontinue use of the product and consider a different nutrient.

For some supplements, and with larger dosages, I recommend splitting your intake into two smaller doses. Your body can only absorb so much of a nutrient at any given time; by taking lesser amounts more frequently, you can thus maximize your absorption, ensuring that your body receives the full advantages of the supplements you take. Be aware that high-fiber diets can also interfere with nutrient absorption; if you are eating a meal that is high in fiber, wait two hours before taking your supplements for best results.

Like all medications, supplements—however natural—can carry certain side effects and risks. They can also interact with specific drugs, causing other health problems. Throughout this book, I have included information on these side effects and contraindications under the heading of "Considerations"—information that will allow you to take the proper precautions in choosing and using supplements. As always, I encourage you to consult with your healthcare practitioner before starting any supplementation regimen; your personal physician will be better able to tailor that regimen to your specific medical status, history, and needs.

OMEGA FATTY ACIDS

Omega fatty acids are essential polyunsaturated fats, meaning that they are not made by your body, but are critical to your body's functioning. When consumed in appropriate amounts, omega fatty acids can fight inflammation, lower "bad" cholesterol, moderate blood pressure, and generally help reduce your risk of cardiovascular disease. Not only do omega fatty acids guard against independent factors of cognitive decline, but they can also directly improve cognition. In addition to consuming omega-3 and omega-6 fatty acids more generally, as directed in Chapter 12, you may want to supplement with a specific omega-3 fatty acid called docosahexaenoic acid (DHA), which is often found alongside another omega-3 fatty acid called eicosapentaenoic acid (EPA).

DHA is actually a structural component of the brain; it is an integral part of brain tissue, and is found in particularly high concentrations in the hippocampus, your memory center. For this reason alone, it's important to make sure that you have adequate supplies of this important fatty acid. More important, studies show that DHA promotes cognition and memory by encouraging the growth of neurons, increasing the rate at which signals are transmitted between them, and generally protecting your brain cells from inflammation and injury.

Low levels of DHA are associated with the development of learning disorders in children and Alzheimer's disease in older populations. Conversely, studies show that subjects who ate DHA-rich fatty fish in greater quantities (or more regularly) decreased their risk of developing mild cognitive impairment between 19 and 75 percent. DHA also seems to help with depression—itself a risk factor for cognitive decline—and with verbal fluency.

DHA supplementation can even help adults that have already developed some form of cognitive decline. One trial showed that by taking DHA supplements, people with age-related memory impairment improved their performance on certain brain fitness tests. Similarly, certain dementia patients who took DHA supplements daily saw significant improvements in their dementia scores. Unfortunately, DHA supplementation has been found to be less effective in patients with Alzheimer's disease. The good news is that with timely supplementation, you may be able to reduce your risk of ever developing this particular form of dementia.

Food Sources of DHA

- Fatty coldwater fish (salmon, trout, mackerel, sardines, herring)
- Seaweed
- Eggs
- Lamb

Recommended Intake

In addition to eating a diet rich in omega fatty acids, most adults would benefit from supplementing with 1,000 milligrams of pharmaceutical-grade omega-3 fatty acids daily. Adults over the age of fifty should increase their daily dose to 2,000 milligrams. Look for omega-3 fatty acid supplements that are 50 percent DHA and 50 percent EPA; this nutrient composition is best for brain and heart health.

Considerations

In doses greater than those recommended above, EPA and DHA can act as blood thinners. If you are already taking a blood thinner, EPA and DHA can augment its effects. Accordingly, restrict your dosage to 1,000 to 2,000 milligrams unless your doctor has directed you to do otherwise.

VITAMINS

Vitamins are substances that occur naturally in both plants and animals. There are two types of vitamins: fat-soluble vitamins, which are stored in the fat cells of your body, and water-soluble vitamins, which are elimi-nated from your body the same day they are ingested. While you can often meet many of your daily vitamin requirements through diet alone, supplementation may be necessary to compensate for any nutrient deple-tion that your food might suffer.

Vitamin A (Beta-carotene)

Vitamin A is a fat-soluble vitamin that is best known for its support of good vision and skin. There are many different types of vitamin A, but the one that is most advantageous for the brain is beta-carotene. Beta-carotene acts as an antoxidant, protecting your brain cells from free radi-cal damage; it also seems to help reduce the risk of cardiovascular disease, an independent risk factor for cognitive decline. In one recent study, test subjects who received 50 milligrams of beta-carotene daily for one year scored significantly higher than subjects who received a placebo on tests that evaluated overall cognitive function and verbal memory. The beta-carotene group also showed a relatively slower rate of age-relat-ed memory decline.

Food Sources

- Orange-yellow vegetables (carrots, squash, and peppers)

- Orange-yellow fruits (cantaloupe, pink grapefruit, apricots)

- Dark leafy greens (kale, spinach, Swiss chard)

Generally speaking, the more intensely colored a fruit or vegetable is, the richer it is in beta-carotene.

Recommended Intake

Adults should take 5,000 to 10,000 International Units (IU) of vitamin A daily. It is not necessary to take an isolated beta-carotene supplement.

Considerations

Excessive vitamin A consumption (over 10,000 IU daily) can turn the skin yellow or orange, and potentially cause liver damage and death. In women, daily intake of even 5,000 IU can increase the risk of hip fracture. If you are taking a high dose of vitamin A each day, have your doctor monitor your calcium and liver enzyme levels. If you smoke, have liver disease, are exposed to asbestos, or are pregnant, consult with your healthcare practitioner before taking vitamin A.

Vitamin B Complex

There are eleven different water-soluble vitamins in the vitamin B complex. Generally speaking, B vitamins help your body transform food into energy; they also help produce red blood cells. B vitamins are also essential for good cognition and memory by helping to stabilize brain chemistry. Certain B vitamins seem to be especially beneficial for your mind:

- **Vitamin B_1 (thiamine)** is necessary for proper nerve function; it helps protect neurons against oxidative stress (free radical damage). It is also used in the synthesis of acetylcholine, your main memory neurotransmitter. Mild thiamine deficiency can lead to cognitive decline; severe thiamine deficiency can cause Wernicke-Korsakoff syndrome, a brain disorder characterized by dementia. Low thiamine levels are also associated with higher incidence rates of Alzheimer's disease; accordingly, studies show that Alzheimer's patients treated with thiamine see improvement in intellectual function.

- **Vitamin B_3 (niacin)** helps guard against heart disease. It lowers LDL ("bad") cholesterol and raises HDL ("good") cholesterol; it decreases triglycerides, fibrinogen (a substance linked to higher production of dangerous blood clots), and lipoprotein A, a marker of cardiovascular risk. It also assists in the production and processing of the important chemicals pregnenolone and serotonin. A study done on people with high cholesterol levels and heart disease showed that niacin not only lowered cholesterol levels, but also improved memory in two-thirds of all test subjects. Studies show that high doses of niacin are also associated with improved memory in subjects who don't have heart disease, too.

- **Vitamin B_6 (pyridoxine)** helps lower your levels of homocysteine, an amino acid that, when elevated, is linked to both cardiovascular disease and cognitive decline. It also helps synthesize various neurotransmitters that are essential for memory.

- **Vitamin B_9 (folic acid or folate)** may also decrease homocysteine levels, and helps metabolize dopamine, a neurotransmitter associated with memory and learning. Low blood levels of folate are associated with increased risk of certain types of dementia, including Alzheimer's disease; severe folate deficiency can even cause a reversible form of dementia. While some initial studies show that folate supplementation can slow cognitive decline, the research is generally inconclusive on the subject.

- **Vitamin B$_{12}$ (cobalamin)** is critical to the functioning of the brain and nervous system. It is necessary for the production of both neurons and neurotransmitters, and helps in energy metabolism. In addition, it helps lower homocysteine levels. B$_{12}$ deficiency is heavily associated with cognitive decline and dementia; by one estimate, it is seen in 23 to 30 percent of all patients with Alzheimer's disease. Some studies have shown that B$_{12}$ supplementation can potentially help reverse cognitive decline as long as there has been no irreparable brain damage; supplementation seems to be most effective when begun within a year of symptom manifestation.

- **Choline** is technically not a vitamin, though it is an essential nutrient associated with the vitamin B complex. Choline is a precursor for acetylcholine, your main memory neurotransmitter—this means that in order for acetylcholine to be synthesized, choline must first be present. Accordingly, people who are deficient in choline have an increased risk of cognitive decline. Studies show that choline supplementation can enhance memory in patients with mild cognitive decline and Alzheimer's disease; the earlier supplementation is initiated, the greater the results seem to be. When outside choline supplementation is warranted, take alpha-glyceryl phosphoryl choline (GPC), the form that is most easily absorbed into your system.

- **Nicotinamide adenine dinucleotide (NAD+)** is a coenzyme—a helper molecule for enzymatic reactions—found in all the cells in your body. NAD+ and its derivative, NADH, are associated with the vitamin B complex, and are critical to energy metabolism and neurotransmitter synthesis. More important, they seem to protect against cell aging and death in the brain; consequently, some scientists believe that NAD+ and NADH not only help buffer the effects of brain damage and disorders, but also play a significant role in learning and memory.

Food Sources

- Brewer's yeast

- Liver and other organ meats

- Dried legumes (lentils, lima beans, black-eyed peas)

- Eggs

- Whole grains, including wheat and rice bran

Recommended Intake

Because the composition of B-complex vitamins varies from brand to brand, take twice daily according to product instructions.

Considerations

Because B vitamins are water soluble and thus are eliminated quickly from your system, it's important to take them at least twice daily. Supplementing with specific B vitamins can cause deficiencies of other B vitamins and other nutrients.

Vitamin E

Vitamin E is actually a group of eight different fat-soluble vitamins that act as powerful antioxidants, protecting your body and brain from damage caused by free radicals. Low vitamin E levels are associated with dementia, in part because vitamin E can be critical to reducing oxidative stress, a condition that contributes to certain types of dementia (see page 73). One study found that almost 60 percent of elderly patients with dementia had low vitamin E blood levels. Some scientists believe that vitamin E supplementation may also reduce cell death in the hippocampus and generally slow the rate at which symptoms of Alzheimer's disease progress.

Food Sources

- Wheat germ

- Sunflower seeds

- Vegetable oils (sunflower seed oil, safflower oil, sesame oil)

- Nuts (almonds, peanuts)

- Green vegetables (spinach, asparagus, broccoli)

Recommended Intake

Take 200 to 400 IU daily.

Considerations

Avoid synthetic forms of vitamin E; always buy natural supplements that contain a combination of different tocopherols and tocotrienols, the two main subgroups of vitamin E. Vitamin E is very safe for use as a supplement. Because vitamin E is a blood thinner, high doses can increase the risk of bleeding in people who are taking drugs that reduce blood clotting. Ferrous sulfate, a common iron compound, destroys vitamin E, and therefore should not be taken with it. Vitamin E should be taken with other antioxidants for best results.

MINERALS

Minerals are inorganic elements that play many important roles in your body, working in combination with vitamins, hormones, enzymes, and other nutrients in order to regulate thousands of biological functions. Because they cannot be synthesized by your body, it is important that you consume adequate amounts of minerals in order to maintain good health. As you will see, minerals are integral to the functioning of your brain and nervous system. Minerals are categorized according to their weight in your body: minerals that make up at least 0.01 percent of your total body weight are deemed macrominerals, and minerals that account for less than that amount are considered trace minerals or microminerals.

Magnesium

Magnesium is a macromineral that acts as a cofactor. That is to say, magnesium binds to and activates over 300 different enzymes, making it an essential ingredient for the majority of the biochemical reactions within your body. Magnesium is best known for its capacity to enable energy production and metabolism at the cellular level, but it is also critical to good brain function. Magnesium helps fight inflammation, enhances the actions of various antioxidants, and helps maintain the integrity and function of nerve cells. While research into magnesium's role in brain function is still under development, at least one initial study indicates that blood concentrations of magnesium are considerably lower in patients with Alzheimer's disease than in non-Alzheimer's subjects.

Moreover, recent studies make it clear that magnesium supplementation can help combat insomnia and cardiovascular disease, two independent risk factors for cognitive decline.

Food Sources

- Kelp
- Nuts (almonds, cashews, pecans, walnuts)
- Whole grains (wheat brain, millet, brown rice)
- Dried fruit
- Dark leafy greens (spinach, Swiss chard, collards)
- Seafood (shrimp, crab, salmon, scallops)
- Legumes

Recommended Intake

Take 200 to 400 milligrams daily.

Considerations

Magnesium citrate, magnesium glycinate, magnesium gluconate, and magnesium lactate are more easily absorbed than magnesium oxide. Diarrhea and other gastrointestinal disturbances may occur if you take more than 600 milligrams of magnesium each day. Severe magnesium toxicity—though rare—can manifest as low blood pressure, nausea, vomiting, muscle weakness, difficulty breathing, or even cardiac arrest.

Zinc

Zinc is a micromineral that acts as a cofactor for 100 different enzymes in the body, enabling many different biochemical reactions. In addition to playing a critical role in protein synthesis and immune function, zinc acts as an antioxidant, guarding against inflammation and free radical damage. Within the brain, zinc seems to regulate communication between neurons and may even assist the processes by which they are generated. As with most nutrients, too much or too little zinc can be harmful to your brain health. As you read in Chapter 7, elevated zinc levels seem to increase the rate at which amyloid plaques—a hallmark of Alzheimer's disease—are formed. Low zinc levels seem to interfere with neurotransmission, particularly within the hippocampus, your memory center. Both low and high zinc levels are associated with higher risk of Alzheimer's disease.

Food Sources of Zinc

- Oysters
- Nuts

- Red meat
- Dairy products

Recommended Intake

Take 25 to 50 milligrams daily.

Considerations

Zinc picolinate and zinc citrate are more easily absorbed by your body than other zinc compounds. It is important to balance zinc and copper for

Top 12 Memory-Enhancing Supplements

Because there are many supplements that can help boost your memory and cognitive function, it can be confusing to know which ones to take. The following is a list of the supplements that doctors most frequently recommend for their capacity to enhance your mental acuity. These supplements have been extensively researched to confirm both their safety and efficacy. As always, you should consult with your personal physician before beginning any supplementation regimen. Treat this list as a jumping-off point to start that conversation.

- Acetyl-L-carnitine
- Alpha-lipoic acid
- Ashwagandha root
- Coenzyme Q_{10}
- EPA/DHA
- Ginkgo

- Huperzine A
- Phosphatidylserine
- Vinpocetine
- Vitamin B complex
- Vitamin E
- Zinc

It's important to remember that a supplement can have different effects in different people. While the supplements above have the most well-established records for enhancing memory and cognition, they might not be the ones that are best for you. Accordingly, this chapter has provided a more comprehensive guide to supplementing for memory enhancement, giving you access to the full range of your options.

optimal absorption. For every ten to fifteen milligrams of zinc, take one milligram of copper. Zinc dosages in excess of those recommended above can cause gastrointestinal disturbances, including nausea, vomiting, loss of appetite, abdominal pain, and diarrhea.

AMINO ACIDS

Amino acids are best known as the building blocks that make up the 40,000 different proteins in your body. But amino acids are also vital for the proper functioning of your brain and nervous system. There are three kinds of amino acid: essential, nonessential, and conditionally essential amino acids. Essential amino acids are those that are important to biological functioning but cannot be made by your body, and thus must be consumed from outside sources. Nonessential amino acids are made by your body; no additional intake is necessary. Under normal circumstances, your body also makes adequate supplies of conditionally essential amino acids. In certain medical situations, however, your body may require additional sources in order to rectify deficiencies that may occur. This section outlines some of the amino acids that have the greatest impact on your memory and mental acuity.

Acetyl-L-Carnitine

Acetyl-L-carnitine is a derivative of the amino acid carnitine. In addition to its function as an antioxidant, acetyl-L-carnitine performs a number of tasks that are beneficial to your cognitive function: it slows the rate at which your neurotransmitter receptors degenerate, increases oxygen availability and respiratory efficiency, and helps convert stored body fat into energy. Acetyl-L-carnitine also acts as a precursor for your main neurotransmitter of memory, acetylcholine; that is, it can be converted into this important neurotransmitter. Acetyl-L-carnitine has also been shown to help reduce your likelihood of developing cardiovascular disease, an independent risk factor for cognitive decline: it lowers LDL ("bad") cholesterol and triglycerides, and it raises HDL ("good") cholesterol.

For all these reasons, many studies have indicated that taking acetyl-L-carnitine supplements improve both short- and long-term memory; it may also enhance mood, mental focus, and energy. In one study focusing on people with mild cognitive impairment, acetyl-L-carnitine was shown to improve memory, attention, verbal fluency, and daily behavior. Another study showed that the benefits of acetyl-L-carnitine are long-lasting: cognitive improvement persisted for thirty days after supplementation was discontinued. Even better, some studies show that acetyl-L-carnitine may even slow the progression of Alzheimer's disease. Clearly, there are significant benefits to adding acetyl-L-carnitine to your daily regimen.

Food Sources

- Meat and poultry
- Whole milk and dairy products
- Avocado
- Asparagus

Recommended Intake

Take 1,000 to 2,000 milligrams daily.

Considerations

Several nutrients can increase the effectiveness of acetyl-L-carnitine, including alpha-lipoic acid, B vitamins, DHA and EPA, phosphatidyl-choline, and phosphatidylserine. Side effects are rare, but can include gastrointestinal disturbances. Agitation, skin rash, and headache may also occur. Occasionally, people who take acetyl-L-carnitine experience a slightly fishy body odor; this can be prevented by taking the vitamin B_2 (riboflavin) at the same time. If you have kidney or liver disease, see your doctor before taking acetyl-L-carnitine.

Carnosine

Not to be confused with carnitine, carnosine is an amino acid that acts as a powerful antioxidant. It helps prevent glycation, a process that results in free radical production and causes signs of aging. Carnosine also helps regulate your body's levels of copper and zinc—two metals that, when possessed in excess, have been linked to the development of dementia. Accordingly, some studies show that carnosine is an effective treatment for Alzheimer's disease, slowing the progression of its symptoms.

Food Sources

Carnosine can be found in beef, chicken, and pork.

Recommended Intake

Take 1,000 to 2,000 milligrams daily.

Considerations

If you have kidney or liver disease, consult with your healthcare practitioner before taking carnosine. When consumed in excess of the recommended intake, carnosine may cause hyperactivity.

Tryptophan

Tryptophan is an essential amino acid that acts as the precursor to serotonin, a neurotransmitter associated with mood and happiness. Commonly known as the chemical in turkey that makes us feel drowsy and contented after Thanksgiving dinner, tryptophan is considered a mood stabilizer and sleep aid. Scientists also link tryptophan and its byproduct, serotonin, to overall cognitive health. One study showed that otherwise healthy patients who consumed a tryptophan-deficient diet experienced temporary impairment of their long-term memory. Another study showed that fasting blood levels of tryptophan tended to be lower in patients with dementia; this may simply be because tryptophan is less easily absorbed than other amino acids.

Food Sources

- Dairy products
- Eggs
- Legumes
- Nuts
- Poultry

Recommended Intake

Take 5 to 50 milligrams daily.

Considerations

If you are taking a selective serotonin reuptake inhibitor (SSRI) or monoamine (MAO) oxidase inhibitor, you should avoid taking tryptophan supplements.

HERBS

For thousands of years, people have harvested plants for their medicinal value. Herbs are a special subset of these healing plants; to this day, many healthcare practitioners recommend herbs as a natural way to achieve optimal health. Herbs have many different healing powers. Some help lower cholesterol and reduce your risk of heart disease, others counteract stress, and still others improve your memory and cognitive function.

Because herbs are "natural," they are commonly believed to be safer than prescription drugs. This is perhaps misleading; as with any dietary supplement, herbs can have serious and harmful effects if not taken with the proper precautions. Further, unlike prescription medications, the quality and contents of many herbal supplements are not regulated by the United States government. Be an informed consumer: carefully read the ingredient list of any supplement you buy, review the considerations provided here, and consult with your doctor before starting any supplement regimen.

Ashwagandha Root (*Withania somnifera*)

Ashwagandha root (*Withania somnifera*) is an herb that is found in India, Pakistan, and Sri Lanka. It is best known for its capacity to improve resistance to emotional and physical stress—a common source for cognitive decline, as you saw in Chapter 4. But ashwagandha also plays several other roles within your brain and nervous system. It stimulates neuron regeneration and repair, and helps maintain proper levels of acetylcholine, your main memory neurotransmitter, by inhibiting the production of acetylcholinesterase, an enzyme that breaks down this important neurotransmitter. It also has antioxidant and anti-inflammatory properties, further protecting your neurons against damage. These characteristics make ashwagandha a useful herb for improving your alertness and memory.

Recommended Intake

In capsule form, ashwagandha can be taken in 500- to 2,000-milligram doses. If preparing the dried root in tea, use three to four ounces daily.

Considerations

May cause gastrointestinal disturbances, including diarrhea, nausea, and vomiting. Do not take ashwagandha root if you are already taking another prescribed cholinesterase inhibitor, such as donepezil (Aricept) or galantamine (Razadyne).

Ginkgo (*Ginkgo biloba*)

Ginkgo (*Ginkgo biloba*) is an herbal extract made from the leaves of the ginkgo tree. Ginkgo's benefits for memory and mental acuity are well-established: it acts as an antioxidant and protects the hippocampus—your memory center—from age-related shrinkage. Ginkgo also encourages the production of acetylcholine (your main memory neurotransmitter) and stimulates the production of additional receptors for serotonin, a neurotransmitter associated with mood and learning. In addition, ginkgo helps protect against cardiovascular disease, an independent risk factor for cognitive decline: it dilates blood vessels and serves as a blood thinner, decreasing blood clotting and improving the circulation of oxygen within your brain and nervous system.

Studies show that ginkgo biloba may prevent age-related decline in both acetylcholine and serotonin receptors on your neurons, helping maintain their sensitivity to neurotransmitters; ginkgo also seems to increase the rate at which neurotransmission occurred. Animal studies indicate that ginkgo may also inhibit the formation of the amyloid plaques associated with Alzheimer's disease and other forms of dementia. For these reasons and others, studies overwhelmingly show that ginkgo supplementation can either stabilize or improve memory and mental acuity in those with mild cognitive impairment or dementia.

Recommended Intake

Take 60 to 120 milligrams daily.

Considerations

Side effects are not common, but can include headaches, nausea, vomiting, or dizziness. Because ginkgo acts as a blood thinner, it should not be used in conjunction with other anticoagulants. Do not take it if you are pregnant or using an MAO inhibitor. If you are taking cyclosporine, papverine, thiazide diuretics, or trazodone, consult with your healthcare practitioner before taking ginkgo.

Grape Seed Extract

Grape seed extract is known for its high concentration of vitamin E and other antioxidants. By one estimate, grape seed extract is twenty times more potent than vitamin E and fifty times more powerful than vitamin C when it comes to fighting free radicals. Furthermore, grape seed extract seems to protect the brain against the formation of amyloid plaques. In addition to preventing inflammation, grape seed extract may also perform other tasks that reduce your risk of developing cardiovascular disease, decreasing high blood pressure (hypertension), lowering LDL ("bad") cholesterol, and discouraging blood clotting.

Recommended Intake

Take 50 to 200 milligrams daily in capsule or tablet form.

Considerations

Side effects are rare, but may include headache, dizziness, and nausea. Because grape seed extract can act as a blood thinner, do not take if you are already using anticoagulants.

Huperzine A

Huperzine A is a compound isolated from the Chinese botanical *Huperzia serrata*. It performs a number of useful functions in the brain: it protects your neurons against toxic levels of the neurotransmitter glutamate, and it inhibits acetylcholinesterase, the enzyme that breaks down acetyl-choline, your main memory neurotransmitter. Because of this character-istics, huperzine A is currently being proposed as a treatment for Alzheimer's disease and other disorders characterized by neurodegener-ation (deterioration of the nerve cells). A recent study conducted by the National Institute of Aging indicated that when taken in large enough doses, huperzine A improved cognitive function and daily behavior in patients with mild to moderate Alzheimer's disease.

Recommended Intake

Take 400 micrograms daily.

Considerations

Side effects are rare, but include gastrointestinal disturbances such as nausea, vomiting, abdominal pain, and diarrhea. Huperzine A may also incur sweating, blurred vision, and increased urination and salivation. Do not take huperzine A if you are already taking another prescribed cholinesterase inhibitor, such as donepezil (Aricept) or galantamine (Razadyne).

Vinpocetine

Vinpocetine is an extract derived from the periwinkle plant. It has sever-al uses within the brain and nervous system. It acts as an anti-inflammatory agent and increases blood circulation within the brain by acting as a blood thinner and dilating (widening) your blood vessels. Vinpocetine also enhances the electrical connectivity of your neural network, increases levels of the neurotransmitter serotonin, and protects your neurons from damage caused by excessive levels of intercellular calcium. Several studies have shown that vinpocetine supplementation improved various aspects of cognitive performance—including attention, concentration, and memory—in patients with dementia.

Recommended Intake

Take 10 to 40 milligrams daily.

Considerations

Side effects are very rare, but can include headaches, chest pains, dizziness, dry mouth, nausea, and skin irritation. Because vinpocetine is a blood thinner, consult with your healthcare practitioner if you are already taking an anticoagulant.

OTHER SUPPLEMENTS

In addition to the vitamins, minerals, and amino acids listed above, there are a number of other supplements that can help you maintain your memory and mental acuity.

Alpha-lipoic Acid

Alpha-lipoid acid, also known as lipoic acid or α-lipoid acid, is a nutrient that is both fat and water soluble, encouraging maximal absorption in the brain. In addition to its antioxidant function, alpha-lipoic acid stimulates the generation of new nerve fibers on your neurons, helping to strengthen memory and slow brain aging. It also acts as a chelating agent, allowing your body to process and remove heavy metals such as iron, copper, and cadmium.

Food Sources

Alpha-lipoic acid is an antioxidant that occurs naturally in a variety of foods; it is usually bound to a substance called lysine that is found in proteins. While data is limited, initial studies indicate that high concentrations of alpha-lipoic acid can be found in organ meats (kidneys, heart, liver) and in certain vegetables, including spinach, broccoli, tomatoes, peas, and Brussels sprouts. Still, none of these foods are adequate as therapeutic sources of alpha-lipoic acid; it would take 100 pounds of spinach to deliver the dose recommended below.

Recommended Intake

Take 100 milligrams daily, in capsule or tablet form.

Considerations

People with diabetes or low blood sugar levels should consult with their healthcare practitioner before taking alpha-lipoic acid, as this supplement can lower blood sugar levels further.

Coenzyme Q_{10} (CoQ_{10})

Coenzyme Q_{10} is a fat-soluble nutrient that is found in many foods and made in nearly all of your body's tissues. Its primary function is to help produce cellular energy, providing your body and brain with the energy they need to run at optimal levels. It also acts as an antioxidant and helps your body regenerate vitamin E.

Food Sources

- Fatty fishes (anchovies, mackerel, salmon, sardine)
- Beef heart
- Broccoli
- Spinach
- Nuts

Recommended Intake

Take 30 to 360 milligrams daily, or as your healthcare practitioner recommends.

Considerations

Do not take more than 100 milligrams daily without express instructions from your healthcare practitioner. If you are taking a blood thinner, consult your doctor before taking CoQ_{10}. Side effects can include digestive disturbances (discomfort, appetite loss, diarrhea, heartburn), insomnia, nausea, and palpitations. Doses greater than 300 milligrams can increase your liver enzymes.

Phosphatidylserine (PS)

Phosphatidylserine (PS) is a phospholipid that occurs naturally in the brain. PS encourages cell-to-cell communication by increasing the production of several important neurotransmitters, including acetylcholine, serotonin, epinephrine, norepinephrine, and dopamine. It also helps protect against stress and fuels the brain by increasing glucose metabolism. Accordingly, studies have shown that PS helps maintain memory in healthy people and improves cognition in people with normal age-related memory impairment. Phosphatidylserine may also help treat the symptoms of certain forms of dementia, including Alzheimer's disease. As with many supplements, for best results, a regimen that includes phosphatidylserine should be initiated before or soon after symptoms of memory loss begin to appear.

Recommended Intake

Take 300 milligrams daily.

Considerations

Studies on phosphatidylserine were predominantly conducted on supplements that had been derived from the brains of cows. Because of the rising incidence of mad cow disease, supplements are now primarily made from soy or cabbage products; the cognitive benefits and risks of these new supplements are yet to be determined.

CONCLUSION

The purpose of this chapter was to provide an overview of the most common supplements used to improve memory and mental acuity. While dietary supplements can provide significant benefits to their consumers, they should be seen as just one part of a larger strategy for memory maintenance and enhancement. For best results, you will need to make certain changes to your lifestyle, as outlined in the rest of Part II. With more physical and mental activity, a healthy diet, better exercise, more sleep, and less stress, nutritional supplements can help you keep your mind sharp and accurate.

Conclusion

Only a few decades ago, people believed that memory loss in the elderly was a natural and unavoidable part of life. Grandma's or grandpa's forgetfulness was certainly a problem, but it could be tolerated—until it began to interfere with their ability to live on their own. Today, however, with an ever-increasing portion of our population reaching the age of sixty-five and beyond, we have come to realize the serious nature of memory loss. Over the last thirty years, billions of dollars have been invested in the study of various memory-robbing illnesses. Great advances have been made in our understanding of these illnesses, but sometimes the research yields more questions than answers. While scientists have been able to identify and isolate specific diseases, and are slowly learning how these diseases work, they have yet to find cures for the most serious forms of memory loss.

On the other hand, as these disorders have been researched, we have also come to realize that through the process of aging, there takes place a "normal" loss of memory and cognitive function. In many cases, though, this loss is not necessarily as normal as it might seem. Instead, this memory loss occurs as the result of a specific cause—a cause that can often be lessened, reversed, or prevented entirely. For all too many people, it is easier to accept the inevitability of age-related problems than it is to do something about it. But for those of you who are reading this book, there is an awareness that losing your memory need *not* be inevitable: you understand that it is within your power not to embrace the "norm."

The material in this book is specifically designed to show you how to preserve your memory and slow cognitive decline—it may even help you get back what you have lost. If your memory loss is caused by a specific problem or condition, Part I will help you figure out what that problem is—and how to fix it. Or, if you are looking for a more general regimen that will help keep your mind in peak condition, Part II will provide you with an appropriate program to adopt and maintain. The important thing is that you maintain this regimen consistently. If you can make the commitment to improve your diet, sleep, stress levels, exercise, and mental activity, you will see results soon enough.

In addition, I have attempted to provide you with the latest findings on the subject of dementia. I know how devastating dementia can be. My own mother suffers the effects of Alzheimer's disease; over the last few years, she has slowly lost a lifetime of precious memories. The work I did in researching my mother's illness became the basis for this book. While there is currently no cure for Alzheimer's disease or any of the other serious forms of memory loss, new treatments are being developed every day. Hope is on the horizon: perhaps even within my lifetime these awful disorders will be eradicated.

You *can* keep your mind sharp and accurate, no matter how old you are. If I can leave you with one message, it is this: take the next step. Whether it is through your faith in God, for someone you love, or because you believe you are the master of your own destiny, you must summon the will to take control of your health. Only you can determine how well or how poorly your mind fares as you age. Use this book as a guide and enjoy great memory and focus for years to come!

Resources

NATURAL MEDICINE SPECIALISTS

To ensure optimal health, it is important to work with a healthcare practitioner who will be take your medical history into account in formulating a personal regimen for you. Below, you'll find two organizations that can lead you to local professionals who specialize in natural and alternative health, nutrition, anti-aging, and metabolic medicine.

American Academy of Anti-Aging Physicians
1801 North Military Trail, Suite 200
Boca Raton, FL 33431
(888) 997-0112
www.a4m.com

Institute for Functional Medicine
505 South 336th Street, Suite 500
Federal Way, WA 98003
(800) 228-0622
(253) 661-3010
www.functionalmedicine.org

DIAGNOSTIC LABORATORIES

The following is a list of diagnostic laboratories that offer tests to evaluate your genetics, hormone and nutrient levels, gastrointestinal function, and heavy metal exposure. These tests can be instrumental in identifying whether you are genetically predisposed to cognitive decline heart disease, or whether heavy metal poisoning, hormonal imbalance, nutritional deficiency, or inflammation is affecting your memory. Before ordering any medical test, consult with your healthcare practitioner.

Age Diagnostic Laboratories
154 Northwest 16th Street
Boca Raton, FL 33432
(877) 983-7863
www.adltests.com

Doctor's Data Laboratory
3755 Illinois Avenue
St. Charles, IL 60174
(800) 323-2784
www.doctorsdata.com

Genova Diagnostic Laboratory
63 Zillicoa Street
Asheville, NC 28801
(800) 522-4762
www.gdx.net

Metametrix Clinical Laboratory
3425 Corporate Way
Duluth, GA 30096
(800) 221-4640 ● (770) 446-5483
www.metametrix.com

NeuroScience, Inc.
373 280th Street
Osceola, WI 54020
(888) 342-7272 ● (715) 755-3995
www.neurorelief.com

Pathways Genomics Corporation
4045 Sorrento Valley Blvd.
San Diego CA, 92121
(877) 505-7374
www.pathway.com

Spectracell Laboratories
10401 Town Park Drive
Houston, TX 77072
(800) 227-5227 ● (713) 621-3101
www.spectracell.com

ZRT Laboratory
8605 Southwest Creekside Place
Beaverton, OR 97006
(866) 600-1635
www.zrtlab.com

PHARMACEUTICAL-GRADE SUPPLEMENTS

Throughout this book, nutritional supplements have been recommended to help alleviate or treat the symptoms of various medical conditions. Below, you'll find a guide to companies that offer high-quality, pharmaceutical-grade supplements. Many of these companies distribute their products only to licensed physicians and compounding pharmacies; their information is provided so that you will be able to locate reliable sources that offer these products near you. As always, consult with your healthcare practitioner before beginning any supplementation regimen.

Designs for Health
2 North Road
East Windsor, CT 06088
(800) 367-4325
www.designsforhealth.com

Douglas Laboratories
112 Technology Drive
Pittsburgh, PA 15275
(800) 245-4440
www.douglaslabs.com

Life Extension
P.O. Box 407189
Fort Lauderdale, FL 33340
(800) 544-4440
www.lef.org

Ortho Molecular Products
1991 Duncan Place
Woodstock, IL 60098
(800) 476-4664 • (815) 337-0089
www.orthomolecularproducts.com

Metagenics
25 Enterprise
Aliso Viejo, CA 92656
(800) 692-9400 • (949) 366-0818
www.metagenics.com

Pain and Stress Center
17579 Frank Madla Road #11
Helotes, TX 78023
(800) 669-2256 • (210) 614-7246
www.painstresscenter.com

MORE INFORMATION ON MEMORY LOSS AND DEMENTIA

The organizations below promote education and research on various forms of cognitive impairment and dementia. They offer comprehensive reviews of current medical knowledge and provide valuable support for the friends and families of people suffering from dementia.

The Alzheimer's Association
225 North Michigan Avenue,
   17th floor
Chicago, IL 60601
(800) 272-3900
www.alz.org

Alzheimer's Foundation of America
322 Eighth Avenue, 7th floor
New York, NY 10001
(866) 232-8484
www.alzfdn.org

**The Association for Fronto-
   temporal Degeneration**
Radnor Station Building 2, Suite 320
290 King of Prussia Road
Radnor, PA 19087

(866) 507-7222 • (267) 514-7221
www.theaftd.com

Lewy Body Dementia Association
912 Killian Hill Road Southwest
Lilburn, GA 30047
(800) 539-9767 • (404) 935-6444
www.lbda.org

The National Institute on Aging
Building 31, Room 5C27
31 Center Drive, MSC 2292
Bethesda, MD 20892
(800) 438-4380
www.nia.nih.gov

BRAIN TRAINING

Based on the growing research on neuroplasticity, a number of national and web-based franchises promise to increase your memory capacity and even your intelligence by teaching you to perform better on certain cognitive tasks. While the research is still inconclusive on the true efficacy of this "brain training," there certainly does not seem to be any harm in engaging in any of these mental activity-boosters—and there may very well be benefits.

CogMed Working Memory Training
200 East Fifth Avenue, Suite 125B
Naperville, IL 60563
(888) 748-3828
www.cogmed.com

Lumosity
153 Kearny Street
San Francisco, CA 94108
www.lumosity.com

Posit Science
77 Geary Street, Suite 303
San Francisco, CA 94108
www.positscience.com

References

Chapter 1: The Brain and Memory Loss

Blennow, K, et al. "Tau protein in cerebrospinal fluid: a biochemical marker for axonal degeneration in Alzheimer disease?" *Mol Chem Neuropathol* 1995; 26(3):231–45.

Boiler, F, et al. "Alzheimer's disease and THA: a review of the cholinergic theory and of preliminary results." *Biomed Pharmacother* 1989; 43(7): 487–91.

Brickman A, and Y Stern. "Aging and Memory in Humans." In *Encyclopedia of Neuroscience*, edited by Larry R. Squire, 175–180. Oxford, United Kingdom: Academic Press, 2009.

Budson, A, and P Solomon. *Memory Loss: A Practical Guide For Clinicians*. Philadelphia: Elsevier/Saunders, 2011.

Davis, K, et al. "Cholinergic markers in elderly patients with early signs of Alzheimer disease," *JAMA* 1999; 281(15):1401–06.

Gauthier, S, et al. "Mild cognitive impairment." *Lancet* 2006; 367:1262–1270.

Graham, Judith. "Coping with Mild Cognitive Impairment," *New York Times*, September 10, 2009. http://newoldage.blogs.nytimes.com/2012/09/10/coping-with-mild-cognitive-impairment/?_r=0

House, E, et al. "Copper abolishes the beta-sheet secondary structure of preformed amyloid fibrils of amyloid-beta." *J Alzheimer's Dis* 2009; 18(4):811–7.

Hung, Y, et al. "Copper in the brain and Alzheimer's disease," *Jour Biol Inorg Chem* 2010; 15(1):61–76.

Lombard, J. "Biomarkers in Neuropsychiatry." Fellowship in Anti-Aging, Regenerative, and Functional Medicine, Module III, Las Vegas, February 28–March 2, 2013.

Markesbery, W. "Oxidative stress hypothesis in Alzheimer's disease." *Free Radic Biol Med* 1997; 23(1):134–47.

Mendez, M, and J Cummings. *Dementia: A Clinical Approach*. Philadelphia: Butterworth-Heinemann, 2003.

National Institute on Aging. "New research illuminates memory loss and early dementia." Last modified April 1, 2009. www.nia.nih.gov/alzheimers/features/new-research-illuminates-memory-loss-and-early-dementia.

National Institute of Neurological Disorders and Stroke. "Dementia: Hope Through Research." Last modified June 26, 2013. www.ninds.nih.gov/disorders/dementias/detail_dementia.htm#2300019213.

Perry, G, et al. "Alzheimer's disease and oxidative stress." *Jour Biomed Biotechnol* 2002; 2(3): 120–3.

Plassman, B, et al. "Prevalence of Dementia in the United States: The Aging, Demographics, and Memory Study." *Neuroepidemiology* 2007; 29(1–2): 125–132.

Raz, N, et al. "Regional brain changes in aging healthy adults: general trends, individual differences, and modifiers." *Cereb Cortex* 2005; 15(11): 1676–1689.

Sherwood, C, et al. "Aging of the cerebral cortex differs between humans and chimpanzees." Proceedings of the National Academy of Sciences of the United States of America 2011; 108(32): 13029–13034.

Small, G. "What we need to know about age-related memory loss." BMJ 2002; 347(7352): 1502–5.

Sonkusare, S, et al. "Dementia of Alzheimer's disease and other neurodegenerative disorders: memantine, a new hope." Pharmacol Res 2005; 51(1):1–17.

Stickgold, R. "Sleep-dependent memory consolidation," Nature 2005; 437(27):1272–8.

Thies, W, et al. "2013 Alzheimer's Disease Facts and Figures," Alzheimer's Dementia 2013; 9(2): 208–45.

Town, T. "Alternative AB immunotherapy approaches for Alzheimer's disease." CNS Neurol Disord Drug Targets 2009; 8(2):114–27.

Walsh, W. Nutrient Power: Heal Your Biochemistry and Heal Your Brain. New York: Skyhorse Publishing, 2012.

Yang, X., et al., "Coordinating to three histidine residues: Cu (II) promotes oligometric and fibrillar amyloid-B peptide to precipitate in a non-B-aggregation way," J Alzheimer's Dis 2009; 18 (4):799–810.

Youngjohn, J, et al. "First-last names and the grocery list selective reminding test: two computerized measures of everyday verbal learning." Arch of Clin Neuropsychology 1991; 6(4): 287–300.

Zhang, Q, et al. "Metabolite-initiated protein misfolding may trigger Alzheimer's disease," Proc Natl Acad Sci 2004; 101(14):4752–7.

Chapter 2: Cardiovascular Disease

Albers, J, et al., "Reduction of lecithin-cholesterol acyltransferase, apolipoprotein D and the Lp(a) lipoprotein with the anabolic steroid stanozolol." BBA: Lipids Lipid Metab 1984; 795(2): 293–6.

Annewieke, W, et al. "Measures of bioavailable serum testosterone and estradiol and their relationships with muscle strength, bone density, and body composition in elderly men." J Clin Endo Metab 2000; 85(9):3276–3282.

Asvold, B, et al. "The association between TSH within the reference range and serum lipid concentrations in a population-based study." Eur J Endocrinol 2007; 156(2):181–6.

Auer, J, et al. "Thyroid function is associated with presence and severity of coronary atherosclerosis." Clin Cardiol 2003; 26(12):569–73.

Ball, P, et al. "Formation, metabolism, and physiologic importance of catecholestrogens." Am J Obstet Gynecol 1990; 163(6):2163–70.

Barrett-Connor, E, et al. "A prospective study of dehydroepiandrosterone sulfate, mortality, and cardiovascular disease." NEJM 1986; 315(24): 1519–24.

Bassil, N, and J Morley. "Late-life onset hypogonadism: a review." Clin Geriatr Med 2010; 26 (2):197–222.

Baum, N, and C Crespi. "Testosterone replacement in elderly men," Geriatrics 2007;62(9):15–8.

Budoff, M, et al. "Effects of hormone replacement on progression of coronary calcium as measured by electron beam tomography." J Women's Health 2005; 14(5):410–7.

Bush, D, et al. "Estrogen replacement reverses endothelial dysfunction in postmenopausal women." Am J Med 1998; 104(6):552–8.

Bush, T. "Cardiovascular mortality and non-contraceptive estrogen use in women: results from the Lipid Research Clinics Program Follow-up Study." Circulation 1987; 75(6):1102–9.

—. "Extraskeletal effects of estrogen and the prevention of atherosclerosis." Osteoporos Int 1991; 2(1):5–11.

Carmody, B, et al. "Progesterone inhibits human infragenicular arterial smooth muscle cell proliferation induced by high glucose and insulin concentrations." J Vasc Surg 2002; 36(4): 833–8.

Caulin-Glaser, T, et al. "Effects of 17ß-estradiol on cytokine-induced endothelial cell adhesion molecule expression." J Clin Invest 1996; 98(1): 36–42.

Chen, F, et al. "Comparison of transdermal and oral estrogen-progestin replacement therapy: effects on cardiovascular risk factors." Menopause 2001; 8(5):347–52.

Chen, J, et al. "Effect of large-dose progesterone on plasma levels of lipids, lipoproteins and apolipoproteins in males." *J Endocrinol Invest* 1986; 9(4):281–5.

Christ-Crain, M, et al. "Elevated C-reactive protein and homocysteine values: cardiovascular risk factors in hypothyroidism? A cross-sectional and double-blind, placebo-controlled trial." *Atherosclerosis* 2003; 166(2):379–86.

Collins, J. *What's Your Menopause Type?* Roseville, CA: Prima Publishing, 2000.

Crook, D, et al. "Pulsatility index in internal carotid artery in relation to transdermal oestradiol and time since menopause." *Lancet* 1991; 338(8771):839–42.

Danesh, J, et al. "Lipoprotein(a) and cardiovascular disease." *Circulation* 2000; 102:1082–5.

Dayas, C, et al. "Effects of chronic oestrogen replacement on stress-induced activation of hypothalamic-pituitary-adrenal axis control pathways." *J Neuroendocrinol* 2000; 12(8):784–4.

Ding, E., et al., "Sex differences of endogenous sex hormones and risk of type 2 diabetes: a systematic review and meta-analysis." *JAMA* 2006; 295(11):1288–99.

Dominguez-Rodriguez, A, et al. "Prognostic value of nocturnal melatonin levels as a novel marker in patients with ST-segment elevation myocardial infarction." *Am J Cardiol* 2006; 97 (8):1162–4.

Dominguez-Rodriguez, A, et al., "Relation of nocturnal melatonin levels to C-reactive protein concentration in patients with ST-segment elevation myocardial infarction." *Am J Cardiol* 2006; 97(1):10–2.

Dubey, R, et al. "Estradiol metabolites inhibit endothelin synthesis by an estrogen receptor-independent mechanism." *Hypertension* 2001; 37(2):640–4.

Duckles, S., et al., "Estrogen and mitochondria: a new paradigm for vascular protection?" *Mol Interv* 2006; 6(1):26–35.

Feldman, H, et al. "Low dehydroepiandrosterone sulfate and heart disease in middle-aged men: cross-sectional results from the Massachusetts Male Aging Study." *Ann Epidemiol* 1998; 8(4):217–28.

Feletou, M, et al. "Endothelial dysfunction: a multifaceted disorder." *Am J Physiol* 2006; 291(3): H985–H1002.

Fernandez-Real, J, et al. "Thyroid function is intrinsically linked to insulin sensitivity and endothelium-dependent vasodilation in healthy euthyroid subjects." *J Clin Endocrinol Metab* 2006; 91(9):3337–43.

Foegh, M, et al. "Estradiol inhibition of arterial neointimal hyperplasia after balloon injury." *J Vasc Surg* 1994; 19(4):722–26.

Franklyn, J, et al. "Thyroid status in patients after acute myocardial infarction." *Clin Sci* 1984; 67:585–90.

Gallagher, P, et al. "Estrogen regulation of angiotensin-converting enzyme mRNA." *Hypertension* 1999; 33(1):323–28.

Grodstein, F, et al. "Postmenopausal hormone therapy and mortality," *NEJM* 1997; 336(25): 1769–76.

Güder, G, et al. "Low circulating androgens and mortality risk in heart failure." *Heart* 2010; 96(7):504–9.

Hak, A, et al. "Subclinical hypothyroidism is an independent risk factor for atherosclerosis and myocardial infarction in elderly women: the Rotterdam Study." *Ann Inter Med* 2000; 132(4):270–8.

Hardiman, P, et al. "Polycystic ovary syndrome and endometrial carcinoma." *Lancet* 2003; 361 (9371):1810–2.

Harman, S, et al. "Male menopause, myth or menace?" *Endocrinologist* 1994; 4(3):212–7.

Henderson, B, et al. "Estrogen replacement therapy and protection from acute myocardial infarction." *Am J Obstet Gynecol* 1988; 159(2): 312–7.

Herbison, A, et al. "Oestrogen modulation of noradrenaline neurotransmission." *Novartis Found Symp* 2000; 230:74–85, discussion 85–93.

Hörner, S, et al. "A statistically significant sex difference in the number of colony-forming cells from human peripheral blood." *Ann Hematol* 1997; 74(6):259–63.

Huber, M, et al. "Post-translational cooperativity of ornithine decarboxylase induction by estrogens and peptide growth factors in human breast cancer cells." *Mol Cell Endocrinol* 1996; 117(2):211–8.

Juan, S, et al. "17ß-estradiol inhibits cyclic strain-induced endothelin-1 gene expression within vascular endothelial cells." *Am J Physiol: Heart Circ Physiol* 2004; 287(3):H1254–H1261.

Kannel, W, et al. "Fibrinogen and the risk of cardiovascular disease." *JAMA* 1987; 258(9): 1183–6.

Karim, R, et al. "Relationship between serum levels of sex hormones and progression of subclinical atherosclerosis in postmenopausal women." *J Clin Endocrinol Metabol* 2008; 93(1): 131–8.

Krasinski, K, et al. "Estradiol accelerates functional endothelial recovery after arterial injury." *Circulation* 1997; 95(7):1768–72.

Kumar, A, et al. "Hypoandrogenaemia is associated with subclinical hypothyroidism in men." *Int J Androl* 2007; 30(1):14–20.

Laragh, J, and M Pecker. "Dietary sodium and essential hypertension: some myths, hopes, and truths." *Ann Intern Med* 1983; 98(5):735–43.

Lerchbaum, E, et al. "High estradiol levels are associated with an increase in mortality in older men referred to coronary angiography." *Explin Endocrinol Diabetes* 2001; 119(8):490–96.

Lewis, D, et al. "Genome and hormones: gender differences in physiology selected contribution: effects of sex and ovariectomy on responses to platelets in porcine femoral veins." *J Appl Physiol* 2001; 91(6):2823–30.

L'Hermite, M, et al. "Could transdermal estradiol + progesterone be a safe postmenopausal HRT? A review." *Maturitas* 2008; 60(3–4): 185–201.

Li, L, et al. "Variant estrogen receptor-c-Src molecular interdependence and c-Src structural requirements for endothelial NO synthase activation." *Proc Natl Acad Sci USA* 2007; 104 (42):16468–73.

Lieberman, E, et al. "Estrogen improves endothelium-dependent flow-mediated vasodilation in postmenopausal women." *Ann of Int Med* 1994; 121(12):936–41.

Losordo, D, et al. "Variable expression of the estrogen receptor in normal and artherosclerotic coronary arteries of premenopausal women." *Circulation* 1994; 89(4):1501–10.

MacGregor, G, et al. "Double-blind randomized crossover trial of moderate sodium restriction in essential hypertension." *Lancet* 1982; 319 (8268): 351–5.

Mackey, R, et al. "Hormone therapy, lipoprotein subclasses, and coronary calcification: the Healthy Women Study." *Arch Intern Med* 2005; 165(5): 510–5.

Maddox, Y, et al. "Endothelium-dependent gender differences in the response of the rat aorta." *J Pharmacol Exp Ther* 1987; 240(2):392–5.

Manson, J, et al. "Estrogen therapy and coronary-artery calcification." *NEJM* 2007; 356(25): 2591–2602.

McCrohon, J, et al, "Effects of hormone replacement therapy on the cardiovascular system." In *Estrogens and Progestogens in Clinical Practice*, edited by Ian Fraser, 711–25. New York: Harcourt Publishers, 2000.

Miller, V, et al. "Sex steroids and endothelial function: translating basic science to clinical practice." *Trends Pharmacol Sci* 2007; 28(6) :263–70.

—. "Vascular actions of estrogens: functional implications." *Pharmacological Reviews* 2008; 60(2): 210–41.

—. "Vascular effects of estrogen and progesterone." In *Estrogens and Progestogens in Clinical Practice*, edited by Ian Fraser, 215–53. New York: Harcourt Publishers, 2000.

Mishra, R, et al. "Metabolite ligands of estrogen receptor-beta reduce primate coronary hyperreactivity." *Am J Physiol: Heart Circ Physiol* 2006; 290(1):H295–H3–3.

Moriarty, K, et al. "Minireview: estrogen receptor-mediated rapid signaling." *Endocrinology* 2006; 147(12):5557–63.

Morley, J. "Androgens and aging." *Maturitas* 2001; 38(1):61–71.

Murakami, S. "Taurine and atherosclerosis." *Amino Acids* 2012.

Nabulsi, A, et al. "Association of hormone-replacement therapy with various cardiovascular risk factors in postmenopausal women." *NEJM* 1993; 328(15):1069–75.

Nedrebø, B, et al. "Plasma total homocysteine levels in hyperthyroid and hypothyroid patients." *Metabolism* 1998; 47(1):89–93.

Nickenig, G, et al. "Estrogen modulates AT1 receptor gene expression in vitro and in vivo." *Circulation* 1998; 97(22):2197–2201.

Nieschlag, E, et al. "Investigation, treatment, and

monitoring of late-onset hypogonadism in males." *J Androl* 2006; 27(2):135–7.

O'Keefe, J, et al. "Estrogen replacement therapy after coronary angioplasty in women." *J Am Coll Cardiol* 1997; 29(1):1–5.

O'Lone, R, et al. "Estrogen receptors alpha and beta mediate distinct pathways of vascular gene expression, including genes involved in mitochondrial electron transport and generation of reactive oxygen species." *Mol Endocrinol* 2007; 21(6):1281–96.

Os, I, et al. "Insulin sensitivity in women with coronary heart disease during hormone replacement therapy." *J Womens Health (Larchmt)* 2005; 14(2):137–45.

Ospina, J, et al. "17ß-estradiol decreases vascular tone in cerebral arteries by shifting COX-dependent vasoconstriction to vasodilation." *Am J Physiol: Heart Circ Physiol* 2003; 285(1): H241–H250.

Otsuki, M, et al. "Progesterone, but not medroxyprogesterone, inhibits vascular cell adhesion molecule-1 expression in human vascular endothelial cells." *Arterioscler Thromb Vasc Biol* 2001; 21(2):243–48.

Philip, K, et al. "Greater antiarrhythmic activity of acute 17ß-estradiol in female than male anaesthetized rates: correlation with Ca2 + channel blockade." *Brit J Pharmacol* 2006; 149(3): 233–42.

Prelevic, C, et al. "The effect of oestrogen and progestogen replacement therapy on systolic flow velocity in healthy postmenopausal women." *Maturitas* 1994; 20(1):37–44.

Proundler, A, et al. "Hormone replacement therapy and serum angiotensin-converting-enzyme activity in postmenopausal women." *Lancet* 1995; 346(8967):89–90.

Puder, J, et al. "Estrogen modulates the hypothalamic-pituitary-adrenal and inflammatory cytokine responses to endotoxin in women." *J Clin Endocrinol Metab* 2001; 86(6):2403–8.

Rajkhowa, M, et al. "Polycystic ovary syndrome: a risk for cardiovascular disease?" *BJOG: Int J Obstet Gynecol* 2000; 107(1):11–8.

Rako, S. "Testosterone deficiency: a key factor in the increased cardiovascular risk to women

following hysterectomy or with natural aging?" *J Women's Health* 1998; 7(7):825–59.

Razvi, S, et al. "The influence of age on the relationship between subclinical hypothyroidism and ischemic heart disease: a metaanalysis." *J Clin Endocrinol Metabol* 2008; 93(8):2998–3007.

Reiter, R, et al. "Melatonin: a novel protective agent against oxidative injury of the ischemic/reperfused heart." *Cardiovasc Res* 2003; 58(1):10–9.

—. "When melatonin gets on your nerves: its beneficial actions in experimental models of stroke," *Exp Biol Med* 2005; 230(2):104–17.

Rizza, R., et al., "Androgen effect on insulin action and glucose metabolism." *Mayo Clin Proc* 2000; 75(Suppl):S61–4.

Rosano, G, et al. "Natural progesterone, but not medroxyprogesterone acetate, enhances the beneficial effect of estrogen on exercise-induced myocardial ischemia in postmenopausal women." *J A Coll Cardiol* 2000; 36(7):2154–9.

Rosengren, A, et al. "Association of psychosocial risk factors with risk of acute myocardial infarction in 11,119 cases and 13, 648 controls in 52 countries (the INTERHEART study): case-control study." *Lancet* 2004; 364(9438):953–62.

Sarrel, P. "Cardiovascular aspects of androgens in women." *Semin Reprod Endocrinol* 1998; 16(2): 1221–28.

Sator, M, et al. "The effect of hormone replacement therapy on carotid arteries: measurement with a high frequency ultrasound system." *Maturitas* 1998; 30(1):63–8.

Seed, M, et al. "The effect of hormone replacement therapy and route of administration on selected cardiovascular risk factors in postmenopausal women." *Fam Pract* 2000; 17(6): 497–507.

Shi, Y, et al. "Adventitial myofibroblasts contribute to neointimal formation in injured porcine coronary arteries." *Circulation* 1996; 94(7):1655–64.

Shufelt, C. "DHEA-S levels and cardiovascular disease mortality in postmenopausal women: results from the National Institutes of Health—National Heart, Lung, and Blood Institute (NHLBI)-sponsored Women's Ischemia Syndrome Evaluation (WISE)." *J Clin Endocrinol Metab* 2010; 85(11):4985–92.

Smith, P. *What You Must Know About Women's Hormones*. Garden City Park, NY: Square One Publishing, 2010.

Soma, M, et al. "Plasma Lp(a) concentration after oestrogen and progestrogen in postmenopausal women." *Lancet* 1991; 337(8741): 612.

Stampfer, M, et al. "Postmenopausal estrogen therapy and cardiovascular disease: ten-year follow-up from the Nurses' Health Study." *NEJM* 1991; 325(11):756–62.

Stevenson, J, et al. "Oral versus transdermal hormone replacement therapy." *Int Jour Fertil Menopausal Stud* 1993; 38(Suppl 1):30–5.

Stirone, C, et al. "Estrogen increases mitochondrial efficiency and reduces oxidative stress in cerebral blood vessels." *Mol Pharmacol* 2005; 68(4):959–65.

Strehlow, K, et al. "Modulation of antioxidant enzyme expression and function by estrogen." *Circ Res* 2003; 93(2):170–7.

Stumpf, W, et al. "The heart: a target organ for estradiol." *Science* 1977; 196(4287):319–21.

Sudhir, K, and P Komesaroff. "Cardiovascular actions of estrogens in men." *J Clin Endocrinol Metab* 1999; 84(10):3411–5.

Suzuki, K, et al. "Endocrine environment of benign prostatic hyperplasia: prostate size and volume correlated with serum estrogen concentration." *Scand J Urol Nephrol* 1995; 29(1):65–8.

Swerdloff, R, et al. "Androgen deficiency and aging in men." *West J Med* 1993; 159(5):579–85.

Talbott, E, et al. "Cardiovascular risk in women with polycystic ovary syndrome." *Obstet Gynecol Clin North Am* 2001; 28(1):111–33.

Tollan, A, et al. "Progesterone reduces sympathetic tone without changing blood pressure or fluid balance in men." *Gynecol Obstet Invest* 1993; 36(4):234–8.

Torkler, S, et al. "Inverse association between total testosterone concentrations, incident hypertension, and blood pressure." *Aging Male* 2011; 14(3):176–82.

Ulloa-Aguirre, A, et al. "Endocrine regulation of gonadotropin glycosylation." *Arch Med Res* 2001; 32(6):520–32.

Vermeulen, A, et al. "Androgens in the aging male." *J Clin Endocrin Metab* 1991; 73(2):221–24.

—. "Estradiol in elderly men." *Aging Male* 2002; 5(2):98–102.

Vitale, C, et al. "Time since menopause influences the acute and chronic effect of estrogens on endothelial function." *Arterioscler Thromb Vasc Biol* 2008; 28(2):348–52.

Wild, S, et al. "Long-term consequences of polycystic ovary syndrome: results of a 31-year study." *Hum Fertil* 2000; 3(2):101–05.

Williams, J, et al. "Short-term administration of estrogen and vascular responses of artherosclerotic coronary arteries." *J Am Coll Cardiol* 1992; 20(2):454–7.

Wu, H. "Coordinated regulation of AIB1 transcriptional activity by sumoylation and phosphorylation." *J Biol Chem* 2006; 281(31): 21848–56.

Wu, Z, et al. "Estrogen regulates adrenal angiotensin AT1 receptors by modulating AT1 receptor translation." *Endocrinology* 2003; 144(7): 3251–61.

Yue, P, et al. "Testosterone relaxes rabbit coronary arteries and aorta." *Circulation* 1995; 91(4): 1154–60.

Chapter 3: Heavy Metal Poisoning

Armstrong, R, et al. "Hypothesis: is Alzheimer's disease a metal-induced immune disorder?" *Neurodegeneration* 1995; 4(1):107–11.

Bains, J, and C Shaw. "Neurodegenerative disorders in humans: the role of glutathione in oxidative stress-mediated neuronal death." *Brain Res Brain Res Rev* 1997; 25(3):335–58.

Barnabei, V, et al. "Plasma homocysteine in women taking hormone replacement therapy: the Postmenopausal Estrogen/Progestin Interventions (PEPI) Trial." *J Women's Health Gend Based Med* 1999; 8(9):1167–72.

Bigazzi, P. "Autoimmunity and heavy metals." *Lupus* 1994; 3(6):449–53.

Boushey, C, et al. "A quantitative assessment of plasma homocysteine as a risk factor for vascular disease." *JAMA* 1995; 274(13):1049–57.

Bush, A. "Copper, zinc, and the metallobiology of Alzheimer's disease." *Alzheimer Dis Assoc Disord* 2003; 17(3):147–50.

Clarkson, T. "The three modern faces of mercury." *Environ Health Perspect* 2002; 110(Suppl 1): 11–23.

Connett, E. "Fluoride's effects on the brain." Fluoride Action Network Pesticides Project submission to National Research Council Committee, April 19, 2004.

Corrigan, F, et al. "Tin and fatty acids in dementia." *Prostaglandins Leukot Essent Fatty Acids* 1991; 43(4):229–38.

Cuajungco, M, and G Lees. "Zinc and Alzheimer's disease: is there a direct link?" *Brain Res Brain Res Rev* 1997; 23(3):219–36.

Flora, S, and P Vidhu. "Chelation in metal intoxication." *Int J Environ Res Public Health* 2010; 7(7):2745–2788.

Fowler, B. "Measuring lead exposure in infants, children, and other sensitive populations." Washington D.C.: National Academy Press, 1993.

Fujiyama, J, et al. "Mechanism of methylmercury efflux from cultured astrocytes." *Biochem Pharmacol* 1994; 47(9):1525–30.

Gibly, R, et al. "Manganese." In *Clinical Environmental Health and Toxic Exposures*, edited by J Sullivan and G Krieger, 930–7. Philadelphia: Lippincott, Williams & Wilkins, 2001.

Godfrey, M, et al. "Apolipoprotein E genotyping as a potential biomarker for mercury neurotoxicity." *J Alzheimer's Dis* 2003; 5(3):189–95.

Hock, C, et al. "Increased blood mercury levels in patients with Alzheimer's disease." *J Neural Transm* 1998; 105(1):59–68.

Hung, Y, et al. "Copper in the brain and Alzheimer's disease." *J Biol Inorg Chem* 2010; 15(1): 61–76.

Hussain, S, et al. "Mercuric chloride-induced reactive oxygen species and its effect on antioxidant enzymes in different regions of rat brain." *J Environ Sci Health* 1997; 32(3):395–409.

Jenner, P. "Oxidative damage in neurodegenerative diseases." *Lancet* 1994; 344(8925):796–8.

LaValle, J. "Toxic Metals and Metabolic Regulation Through Chelation." Fellowship in Anti-Aging, Regenerative, and Functional Medicine. Boca Raton, FL. February 18–20, 2011.

Lohr, J, and J Browning. "Free radical involvement in neuropsychiatric illness." *Psychopharmacol Bull* 1995; 31(1):159–65.

McGuire, T. "Chronic mercury poisoning and mercury detoxification." *Townsend Letter* June, 2007: 96–105.

Mikhailets, N, et al. "Thyroid function during prolonged exposure to fluorides." *Probl Endokrinol* 1996; 42:6–9.

Mutter, J, et al. "Alzheimer disease: mercury as pathogenetic factor and apolipoprotein E as a moderator." *Neuro Endocrinol Lett* 2004; 25(5): 331–9.

National Research Council. "Toxicological Effects of Methylmercury." Washington, DC: National Academies Press, 2000.

Navas-Acien, A, et al. "Arsenic exposure and type 2 diabetes: a systematic review of the experimental and epidemiological evidence." *Environ Health Perspect* 2006; 114(5):641–8.

—. "Lead exposure and cardiovascular disease—a systematic review." *Environ Health Perspect* 2007; 115(3):472.

Nick, G. "Addressing mercury bioaccumulation with whole foods." *Townsend Letter* June 2007, 58–62.

Null, G, and M Feldman. "Stop fluoridation now: a new research on fluoride's brain and thyroid toxicity." *Townsend Letter* April 2005; 256–61.

Olivieri, G, et al. "Mercury induces cell cytotoxicity and oxidative stress and increases beta-amyloid secretion and tau phosphorylation in SHSY5Y neuroblastoma cells." *J Neurochem* 2000; 74(1):231–6.

Ong, W, and Farooqui A. "Iron, neuroinflammation, and Alzheimer's disease." *J Alzheimer's Dis* 2005; 8(2):183–200.

Ou, P, et al. "Thioctic (lipoic) acid: a therapeutic metal-chelating antioxidant?" *Biochem Pharmacol* 1995; 50(1):123–26.

Park, S, et al. "Low-level lead exposure, metabolic syndrome, and heart rate variability: the VA Normative Aging Study." *Environ Health Perspect* 2006; 114(11):1718–24.

Pendergrass, J. "The toxic effects of mercury on CNS proteins—similarity to observations in Alzheimer's disease." Paper presented at International Academy of Oral Medicine and Toxicology symposium, March, 1997.

Perlingeiro, R, and M Queiroz. "Polymorphonuclear phagocytosis and killing in workers exposed to inorganic mercury." *Int J Immunopharmacol* 1994; 16(12):1011–17.

Perrin-Nadif, R. "Catalase and superoxide dismutase activities as biomarkers of oxidative stress in workers exposed to mercury vapors." *J Toxicol Environ Health* 1996; 48(2):107–20.

Perry, T, et al. "Parkinson's disease: a disorder due to nigral glutathione deficiency?" Neurosci Lett 1982; 33(3):305–10.

Rönnbäck, L, and E Hansson. "Chronic encephalopathies induced by mercury or lead: aspects of underlying cellular and molecular mechanisms." *Brit J Int Med* 1992; 49(4):233–40.

Schafer, J, et al. "Blood lead is a predictor of homocysteine levels in a population-based study of older adults." *Environ Health Perspect* 2005; 113(1):31–35.

Shenker, B, et al. "Immunotoxic effects of mercuric compounds on human lymphocytes and monocytes. II. Alterations in cell viability." *Immunopharmacol Immunotoxicol* 1992; 14(3):555–77.

Shivarajashankara, Y, et al. "Brain lipid peroxidation and antioxidant systems of young rats in chronic fluoride intoxication." *Fluoride* 2002; 35(3):197–203.

Smith, P. *What You Must Know About Vitamins, Minerals, Herbs, and More.* Garden City Park, NY: Square One Publishing, 2008.

Stokinger, H. "The metals." In *Patty's Industrial Hygiene and Toxicology*, edited by G and F Clayton, 1687–1728. New York: Wiley Interscience, 1981.

Sullivan, J. "Review of organ system toxicology: pulmonary toxicology and neurotoxicology." Paper presented at meeting of Fellowship in Anti-Aging, Regenerative, and Functional Medicine, Module XII, Boca Raton, Florida, February 18–20, 2011.

Takeda, A. "Manganese action in brain function." *Brain Res Brain Res Rev* 2003; 41(1):79–87.

Thompson, C, et al. "Regional brain trace-element studies in Alzheimer's disease." *Neurotoxicology* 1988; 9(1):1–7.

Travieso, R, et al. "Heavy metal removal by microalgae." *Bull Environ Contam Toxicol* 1999; 62(2):144–51.

Wentz, M. *A Mouth Full of Poison: The Truth About Mercury Amalgam Fillings.* Rosarito Beach, Baja California: Medicis, 2004.

Xiang, Q, et al. "Effect of fluoride in drinking water in children's intelligence." *Fluoride* 2003; 36(2):84–94.

Yee, S, and B Choi. "Oxidative stress in neurotoxic effects of methylmercury poisoning." *Neurotoxicology* 1996; 17(1):17–26.

Yip, L, et al. "Arsenic." In *Clinical Environmental Health and Toxic Exposures*, edited by J Sullivan and G Krieger, 858–66. Philadelphia: Lippincott, Williams & Wilkins, 2001.

Chapter 4: Hormonal Imbalance

Abbatecola, A, et al. "Postprandial plasma glucose excursions and cognitive functioning in aged type 2 diabetics." *Neurology* 2006; 67(2): 235–40.

Adams, J. "Bound to work: the free hormone hypothesis revisited." *Cell* 2005; 122(5):647–9.

Aisen, P. "Anti-inflammatory therapy for Alzheimer's disease: implications of the prednisone trial." *Acta Neurol Scand* 2000; 176(Suppl):85–9.

Akwa, Y, et al. "Neurosteroids: biosynthesis, metabolism, and function of pregnenolone and dehydroepiandrosterone in the brain." *J Steroid Biochem Mol Biol* 1991; 40(1–3):71–81.

Alexander, G, et al. "Androgen-behavior correlations in hypogonadal men and eugonadal men." *Horm Behav* 1998; 33(2):85–94.

Alzoubi, K, et al. "Levothyroxine restores hypothyroidism-induced impairment of LTP of hippocampal CA1: electrophysiological and molecular studies." *Exp Neurol* 2005: 195(2): 330–41.

Andreassen, T, "The role of plasma-binding proteins in the cellular uptake of lipophilic vitamins and steroids." *Horm Metab Res* 2006; 38(4):279–90.

Annweiler, C, et al. "Dietary intake of vitamin D and cognition in older women: a large population-based study." *Neurology* 2010; 75(20): 1810–6.

Arboleda, G, et al. "Insulin-like growth factor-1-depdendent maintenance of neuronal metabolism through the phosphatidylinositol 3-kinase-

Akt pathway is inhibited by C2-ceramide in CAD cells." *Eur J Neurosci* 2007; 25(10):3030–8.

Asthana, S, et al. "Cognitive and neuroendocrine response to transdermal estrogen in postmenopausal women with Alzheimer's disease: results of a placebo-controlled, double-blind, pilot study." *Psychoneuroendocrinology* 1999; 24(6): 657–78.

Ballmaier, M, et al. "Hippocampal morphology and distinguishing late-onset from early-onset elderly depression." *Am J Psychiatry* 2008; 165(2):229–37.

Barrett-Conner, E, and D Kritz-Silverstein. "Estrogen replacement therapy and cognitive function in older women." *JAMA* 1993; 269(20): 2637–41.

Bassil, N, and J Morley. "Endocrine aspects of healthy brain aging." In *Healthy Brain Aging: Evidence Based Methods to Preserve Brain Function and Prevent Dementia*, edited by A Desai, 57–74. New York: Elsevier, 2010.

Bernal, J. "Thyroid hormones and brain development." *Vitam Horm* 2005; 71:95–122.

Biessels, G, et al. "Risk of dementia in diabetes mellitus: a systematic review." *Lancet Neurol* 2006; 5(1):64–74.

Bob, P, and P Fedor-Freybergh. "Melatonin, consciousness, and traumatic stress." *J Pineal Res* 2008; 44(4):341–7.

Bourre, J. "Effects of nutrients (in food) on the structure and function of the nervous system: update on dietary requirements for brain. Part I: micronutrients." *J Nutr Health Aging* 2006; 10(5): 377–85.

Bowen, R, et al. "An association of elevated serum gonadotropin elevated serum gonadotropin concentrations and Alzheimer's disease?" *J Neuroendocrinol* 2000; 12(4):351–4.

Brewer, L, et al. "Vitamin D hormone confers neuroprotection in parallel with downregulation of L-type calcium channel expression in hippocampal neurons." *J Neurosci* 2001; 21(1): 98–108.

Buell, J, and B Dawson-Hughes. "Vitamin D and neurocognitive dysfunction: preventing 'D'ecline?" *Mol Aspects Med* 2008; 29(6):415–22.

Burns, J, et al. "Peripheral insulin and brain structure in early Alzheimer disease." *Neurology* 2007; 69(11):1094–1104.

Caldwell, J, and G Jirikowski. "Sex hormone binding globulin and aging." *Horm Metab Res* 2009; 41(3):173–82.

Carpi, M. "Stress: It's worse than you think." *Psychology Today*, Jan 1, 1996. www.psychologytoday.com/articles/199601/stress-its-worse-you-think.

Centers for Disease Control and Prevention and the Alzheimer's Association. *The Healthy Brain Initiative: A National Public Health Road Map to Maintaining Cognitive Health*. Chicago, IL: Alzheimer's Association, 2013.

Cherrier, N, et al. "Cognitive changes associated with supplementation of testosterone or dihydrotestosterone in mildly hypogonadal men: a preliminary report." *J Androl* 2003; 24(4): 568–76.

—. "Testosterone improves spatial memory in men with Alzheimer disease and mild cognitive impairment," *Neurology* 2005; 64(12):2063–8.

Cholerton, B, "Insulin resistance and pathological brain ageing." *Diabet Med* 2011; 28(12): 1463–75.

Chu, L, et al. "Bioavailable testosterone is associated with a reduced risk of amnestic mild cognitive impairment in older men." *Clin Endocrinol* 2008; 68(4):589–98.

Chubb, S, et al. "Lower sex hormone-binding globulin is more strongly associated with metabolic syndrome than lower total testosterone in older men: the Health in Men Study." *Eur J Endocrinol* 2008; 158(6):785–92.

Compton, J, et al. "HRT and its effect on normal ageing of the brain and dementia." *Br J Clin Pharmacol* 2001; 52(6):647–53.

Craft, S, et al. "Intranasal insulin therapy for Alzheimer disease and amnestic mild cognitive impairment: a pilot clinical trial." *Arch Neurol* 2012; 69(1):29–38.

De Quervain, D, et al. "Glucocorticoid-related genetic susceptibility for Alzheimer's disease." *Hum Mol Genet* 2004; 13(1):47–52.

Desai, A, editor. *Healthy Brain Aging: Evidence Based Methods to Preserve Brain Function and Prevent Dementia*. New York: Elsevier, 2010.

Desouza, L, et al. "Thyroid hormone regulates hippocampal neurogenesis in the adult rat brain." *Mol Cell Neurosci* 2005; 29(3):414–26.

Dhamoon, M, et al. "Intranasal insulin improves cognition and modulates beta-amyloid in early AD." *Neurology* 2009; 72(3):292–3.

Di Paolo, T. "Modulation of brain dopamine transmission by sex steroids." *Rev Neurosci* 1994; 5(1):27–41.

Drake, E, et al. "Associations between circulating sex steroid hormones and cognition in normal elderly women." *Neurology* 2000; 54(3): 599–603.

Drummond, E, et al. "Androgens and Alzheimer's disease." *Curr Opin Endocrinol Diabetes Obes* 2009; 16(3):254–9.

Duff, S, and E Hampson. "A beneficial effect of estrogen on working memory in postmenopausal women taking hormone replacement therapy." *Horm Behav* 2000; 38(4):262–76.

Duka, T, et al. "The effects of 3-week estrogen hormone replacement on cognition in elderly healthy females." *Psychopharmacol* 2000; 149(2): 129–39.

Ehninger, D, et al., "Paradoxical effects of learning the Morris water maze on adult hippocampal neurogenesis in mice may be explained by a combination of stress and physical activity." *Genes Brain Behav* 2006; 5(1):29–39.

English, K, et al. "Men with coronary artery disease have lower levels of androgens than men with normal coronary angiograms." *Eur Heart J* 2000; 21(11):890–4.

Farr, S, et al. "DHEAS improves learning and memory in aged SAMP8 mice but not in diabetic mice." *Life Sci* 2004; 75(23):2775–85.

Fewlass, D, et al. "Obesity-related leptin regulates Alzheimer's Abeta." *FASEB J* 2004; 18(15): 1870–8.

Fillit, H, et al. "Observation in a preliminary open trial of estradiol therapy for senile dementia—Alzheimer's type." *Psychoneuroendocrinology* 1986; 11(3):337–45.

Flaherty, J, et al. "Delirium is a serious and under-recognized problem: why assessment of mental status should be the sixth vital sign." *J Am Med Dir Assoc* 2007; 8(5):273–5.

—. "The development of a mental status sign for use across the spectrum of care." *J Am Med Dir Assoc* 2009; 10(6):379–80.

Flood, J, et al. "Age-related decrease of plasma testosterone in SAMP8 mice: replacement improves age-related impairment of learning and memory." *Physiol Behav* 1995; 57(4):669–73.

—. "Characteristics of learning and memory in streptozocin-induced diabetic mice." *Diabetes* 1999; 39(11):1391–8.

Forti, P, et al. "Serum thyroid-stimulating hormone as a predictor of cognitive impairment in an elderly cohort." *Gerontology* 2012; 58(1):41–9.

Fukui, M, and N Nakamura. "Bone and men's health. Association between serum testosterone and bone mineral density in patients with diabetes." *Clin Calcium* 2010; 20(2):206–11.

Funahashi, H, et al. "Distribution, function, and properties of leptin receptors in the brain." *Int Rev Cytol* 2003; 224:1–27.

Gangar, K, et al. "Pulsatility index in internal carotid artery in relation to transdermal oestradiol and time since menopause." *Lancet* 1991; 338(8771):839–42.

Garcia-Segura, L, et al. "Synaptic remodeling in arcuate nucleus after injection of estradiol valerate in adult female rats." *Brain Res* 1986; 366(1–2):131–5.

Garcion, E, et al. "New clues about vitamin D functions in the nervous system." *Trends Endocrinol Metab* 2002; 13(3):100–5.

Gerges, N, and K Alkadhi. "Hypothyroidism impairs late LTP in CA1 region but not in dentate gyrus of the intact rat hippocampus: MAPK involvement." *Hippocampus* 2004; 14(1):40–5.

Gibbs, R, and R Gabor. "Estrogen and cognition: applying preclinical findings to clinical perspectives." *J Neurosci Res* 2003; 74(5):637–43.

Gillett, M, et al. "Relationship between testosterone, sex hormone binding globulin, and plasma amyloid beta peptide 40 in older men with subjective memory loss or dementia." *J Alzheimer's Dis* 2003; 5(4):267–9.

Goodman, Y, et al. "Estrogen attenuates and corticosterone exacerbates excitotoxicity, oxidative injury, and amyloid beta-peptide toxicity in hippocampal neurons." *J Neurochem* 1996; 66(5):1836–44.

Gorwood, P, et al. "Toxic effects of depression on brain function: impairment of delayed recall and the cumulative length of depressive disorder in a large sample of depressed outpatients." *Am J Psychiatry* 2008; 165(6):731–9.

Gouras, G, et al. "Testosterone reduces neuronal secretion of Alzheimer's beta-amyloid peptides." *Proc Nat Acad Sci USA* 2000; 97(3): 1202–5.

Grimley, E, et al. "Dehydroepiandrosterone (DHEA) supplementation for cognitive function in healthy elderly people." *Cochrane Database Syst Rev* 2006; 4:CD006221.

Grunstein, R, et al. "Neuroendocrine dysfunction in sleep apnea: reversal by continuous positive airways pressure therapy." *J Clin Endocrinol Metab* 1989; 68(2):352–8.

Haren, M, et al. "Lower serum DHEAS levels are associated with a higher degree of physical disability and depressive symptoms in middle-aged to older African American women." *Maturitas* 2007; 57(4):347–60.

Harman, S, and M Blackman. "Male menopause, myth or menace?" *Endocrinologist* 1994; 4(3):212–7.

Harvey, J. "Leptin: a multifaceted hormone in the central nervous system." *Mol Neurobiol* 2003; 28(3):245–58.

Harvey, J, et al. "Leptin: a potential cognitive enhancer?" *Biochem Soc Trans* 2005; 33(Pt 5):1029–32.

Hassing, L, et al. "Diabetes mellitus is a risk factor for vascular dementia, but not for Alzheimer's disease: a population-based study of the oldest old." *Int Psychogeriatr* 2002; 14(3): 239–48.

—. "Type 2 diabetes mellitus contributes to cognitive decline in old age: a longitudinal population-based study." *J Int Neuropsychol Soc* 2004; 10(4):599–607.

Hautanen, A. "Synthesis and regulation of sex hormone-binding globulin in obesity." *Int J Obes Relat Metab Disord* 2000; 24(Supp 2): S64–70.

He, X, et al. "Functional magnetic resource imaging assessment of altered brain function in hypothyroidism during working memory processing." *Eur J Endocrinol* 2011; 164(6):951–9.

Henderson, V. "Estrogen replacement therapy for the prevention and treatment of Alzheimer's disease." *CNS Drugs* 1997; 5:343–51.

—. "Postmenopausal hormone therapy and Alzheimer's disease risk: interaction with age." *J Neurol Neurosurg Psychiatry* 2005; 76(1):103–5.

Henderson, V, et al. "Cognitive skills associated with estrogen replacement in women with Alzheimer's disease." *Psychoneuroendocrinology* 1996; 21(4):421–30.

—. "Estrogen replacement therapy in older women. Comparisons between Alzheimer's disease cases and nondemented control subjects." *Arch Neurol* 1994; 51(9):896–900.

Hogervorst, E, et al. "Low free testosterone is an independent risk factor for Alzheimer's disease." *Exp Gerontol* 2004; 39(11–12):1633–9.

—. "The nature of the effect of female gonadal hormone replacement therapy on cognitive function in postmenopausal women: a meta-analysis." *Neuroscience* 2000; 101(3):485–512.

—. "Serum total testosterone is lower in men with Alzheimer's disease." *Neuro Endocrinol Lett* 2001; 22(3):163–8.

Holden, K, et al. "Serum leptin level and cognition in the elderly: findings from the Health ABC study." *Neurobiol Aging* 2009; 30(9):1483–9.

Irie, F, et al. "Enhanced risk for Alzheimer disease in persons with type 2 diabetes and APOE ε4: The Cardiovascular Health Study Cognition Study." *Arch Neurol* 2008; 65(1):89–93.

Irving, A, et al. "Leptin enhances NR2B-mediated N-methyl-D-aspartate responses via a mitogen-activated protein kinase-dependent process in cerebellar granule cells." *Neuroscience* 2006; 138(4):1137–48.

Isidori, A, et al. "Leptin and aging: correlation with endocrine changes in male and female healthy adult populations of different body weights." *J Clin Endocrinol Metab* 2000; 85(5): 1954–62.

Janowsky, J, et al. "Sex steroids modify working memory." *J Cogn Neurosci* 2000; 12(3):407–14.

Joëls, M, et al. "Learning under stress: How does it work?" *Trends Cogn Sci* 2006; 10(4):152–8.

Johnson, L, et al. "The influence of thyroid function on cognition in a sample of ethnically diverse, rural-dwelling women: a project FRONTIER study." *J Neuropsychiatry Clin Neurosci* 2011; 23(2):219–22.

Jorde, R, et al. "Neuropsychological function in relation to serum parathyroid hormone and serum 25-hydroxyvitamin D levels: The Tromsø Study." *J Neurol* 2006; 253(4):464–70.

Kalueff, A, and P Tuohimaa. "Neurosteroid hormone vitamin D and its utility in clinical nutrition." *Curr Opin Clin Nutr Metab Care* 2007; 10(1):12–19.

Kampen, D, and B Sherwin. "Estrogen use and verbal memory in healthy postmenopausal women." *Obstet Gynecol* 1994; 83(6):979–83.

Karlamangla, A, et al. "Increase in epinephrine excretion is associated with cognitive decline in elderly men: MacArthur Studies of Successful Aging." *Psychoneuroendocrinology* 2005; 30(5): 453–60.

Kawas, C, et al. "A prospective study of estrogen replacement therapy and the risk of developing Alzheimer's disease in the Baltimore Longitudinal Study of Aging." *Neurology* 1996; 48(6):1517–21.

Kronenberg, H, et al, editors. *Williams Textbook of Endocrinology.* New York: Elsevier, 2008.

Landfield, P, and L Cadwallader-Neal. "Long-term treatment with calcitrol (1,25 (OH) 2 vit D3) retards a biomarker of hippocampal aging in rats." *Neurobiol Aging* 1998; 19(5):469–77.

LeBlanc, E, et al. "Hormone replacement therapy and cognition: systemic review and meta-analysis." *JAMA* 2001; 285(11):1489–99.

Lee, B, et al. "Associations of salivary cortisol with cognitive function in the Baltimore Memory Study." *Arch Gen Psychiatry* 2007; 64(7):810–8.

Lee, M, and J Chodosh. "Dementia and life expectancy: what do we know?" *J Am Med Dir Assoc* 2009; 10(7):446–71.

Lehmann, D, et al. "The vitamin D receptor gene is associated with Alzheimer's disease." *Neurosci Lett* 2011; 504(2):79–82.

Levin, E. "Integration of the extranuclear and nuclear actions of estrogen." *Mol Endocrinol* 2005; 19(8):1951–9.

Li, C, et al. "Association of testosterone and sex hormone binding globulin with metabolic syndrome and insulin resistance in men." *Diabetes Care* 2010; 33(7):1618–24.

Li, X, et al. "Impairment of long-term potentia-

tion and special memory in leptin receptor-deficient rodents." *Neuroscience* 2002; 111(3): 607–15.

Llewellyn D, et al. "Vitamin D and cognitive impairment in the elderly U.S. population." *J Gerontol A Biol Sci Med Sci* 2011; 66(1):59–65.

López-Jaramillo, P, and E Terán. "Improvement in functions of the central nervous system by estrogen replacement therapy might be related with an increased nitric oxide production." *Endothelium* 1999; 6(4):263–6.

Luchsinger, J, et al. "Hyperinsulinemia and risk of Alzheimer disease." *Neurology* 2004; 63(7): 1187–92.

Luine, V. "Estradiol increases choline acetyltransferase activity in specific basal forebrain nuclei and projection areas of female rats." *Experimental Neurology* 1985; 89(2):484–90.

Luine, V, and B McEwen. "Effect of estradiol on turnover of type A monamine oxidase in brain." *J Neurochem* 1977; 28(6):1221–7.

Liune, V, et al. "Immunochemical demonstration of increased choline acetyltransferase concentration in rat prepoptic area after estradiol administration." *Brain Res* 1980; 19(1):273–7.

Lupien, S, et al. "The modulatory effects of corticosteroids on cognition: studies in young human populations." *Psychoneuroendocrinology* 2002; 27(3):401–16.

MacKnight, C, et al. "Diabetes mellitus and the risk of dementia, Alzheimer's disease, and vascular cognitive impairment in the Canadian Study of Health and Aging." *Dement Geriatr Cogn Disord* 2002; 14(2):77–83.

Maurizi, C, et al. "The mystery of Alzheimer's disease and its prevention by melatonin." *Med Hypothesis* 1995; 45(4):339–40.

Mayo, W, et al. "Individual differences in cognitive aging: implication of pregnenolone sulfate." *Prog Neurobiol* 2003; 71(1):43–8.

—. "Pregnenolone sulfate enhances neurogenesis and PSA-NCAM in young and aged hippocampus." *Neurobiol Aging* 2005; 26(1):103–14.

Mazza, A, and J Morley. "Update on diabetes in the elderly and the application of current therapeutics." *J Am Med Dir Assoc* 2007; 8(8):489–92.

McCann, J, and B Ames. "Is there convincing biological or behavioral evidence linking vitamin D deficiency to brain dysfunction?" *FASEB J* 2008; 22(4):981–1001.

McEwen, B. "Physiology and neurobiology of stress and adaptation: central role of the brain." *Physiol Rev* 2007; 87(3):873–904.

—. "Protective and damaging effects of stress mediators: central role of the brain." *Dialogues Clin Neurosci* 2006; 8(4):367–81.

McGrath, J, et al. "No association between serum 25-hydroxyvitamin D3 level and performance on psychometric tests in NHANES III." *Neuroepidemiology* 2007; 29(1–2):49–54.

McKeever, W, and R Deyo. "Testosterone, dihydrotestosterone and spatial task performance of males." *Bull Psychonom Soc* 1990; 28(4):305–8.

Menéndez, E, et al. "Glucose tolerance and plasma testosterone concentrations in men. Results of the Asturias Study." *Endocrinol Nutr* 2001; 58(1):3–8.

Messinger-Rapport, B, et al. "Clinical update on nursing home medicine: 2008." *J Am Med Dir Assoc* 2008; 9(7):460–75.

Meston, N, et al. "Endocrine effects of nasal continuous positive airway pressure in male patients with obstructive sleep apnea." *J Intern Med* 2003; 254(5):447–54.

Middleton, L, and K Yaffe. "Promising strategies for the prevention of dementia." *Arch Neurol* 2009; 66(10):1210–5.

Moffat, S. "Effects of testosterone on cognitive and brain aging in elderly men." *Ann NY Acad Sci* 2005; 1055:80–92.

Moffat, S, et al. "Free testosterone and risk for Alzheimer disease in older men." *Neurology* 2004; 62(2):188–93.

Moncada, S, et al. "The L-arginine nitric oxide pathway." *NEJM* 1993; 329(27):2002–12.

Montero-Pedrazuela, A, et al. "Modulation of adult hippocampal neurogenesis by thyroid hormones: implications in depressive-like-behavior." *Mol Psychiatry* 2006; 11(4):361–71.

Mooradian, A, et al. "Cortical function in elderly non-insulin dependent diabetic patients. Behavioral and electrophysiologic studies." *Arch Intern Med* 1988; 148:2369–72.

Morali, G, et al. "Neuroprotective effects of

progesterone and allopregnanolone on long-term cognitive outcome after global cerebral ischemia." *Restor Neurol Neurosci* 2011; 29(1):1–15.

Morgan, C, et al. "Relationships among plasma dehydroepiandrosterone sulfate and cortisol levels, symptoms of dissociation, and objective performance in humans exposed to acute stress." *Arch Gen Psychiatry* 2004; 61(8):819–25.

—. "Relationships among plasma dehydroepiandrosterone and dehydroepiandrosterone sulfate, cortisol, symptoms of dissociation, and objective performance in humans exposed to underwater navigation stress." *Biol Psychiatry* 2009; 66(4):334–40.

Morley, J. "Hormones and the aging process." *J Am Geriatr Soc* 2003; 51(7 Suppl):S333–7.

—. "Testosterone and behavior." *Clin Geriatr Med* 2003; 19(3):605–16.

Morley, J, et al. "Evaluation of assays available to measure free testosterone." *Metabolism* 2002; 51(5):554–9.

—. "Longitudinal changes in testosterone, luteinizing hormone, and follicle-stimulating hormone in healthy older men." *Metabolism* 1997; 46(4):410–3.

—. "Potentially predictive and manipulable blood serum correlates of aging in the healthy human male: progressive decreases in bioavailable testosterone, dehydroepiandrosterone sulfate, and the ratio of insulin-like growth factor 1 to growth hormone." *Pro Natl Acad Sci USA* 1997; 94(14):7537–42.

Morreale de Escobar, G, et al. "Is neuropsychological development related to maternal hypothyroidism or to maternal hypothyroxinemia?" *J Clin Endocrinol Metab* 2000; 85(11):3975–87.

Munshi, M, et al. "Cognitive dysfunction is associated with poor diabetes control in older adults." *Diabetes Care* 2006; 29(8):1794–9.

Näsman, B, et al, "Abnormalities in adrenal androgens, but not of glucocorticoids, in early Alzheimer's disease." *Psychoneuroendocrinlogy* 1995; 20(1):83–94.

Nikezic, G, et al. "17 beta-estradiol in vitro affects Na-dependent and depolarization-induced Ca2+ transport in rat brain synaptosomes." *Experimentia* 1996; 52(3):217–20.

Ohkura, T, et al. "An open trial of estrogen therapy for dementia of the Alzheimer type in women." In *Modern Management of the Menopause. Proceedings of the VII International Congress on the Menopause*, edited by G Berg, 315–33. New York: Parthenon Publishing Group 1993.

Ohrvall, U, et al. "Surgery for sporadic primary hyperparathyroidism in the elderly." *World J Surg* 1994; 18(4):612–8.

Olivieri, G, et al. "Melatonin protects SHSY5Y neuroblastoma cells from cobalt-induced oxidative stress, neurotoxicity, and increased beta-amyloid secretion." *J Pineal Res* 2001; 31:320–25.

O'Malley, D, et al. "Leptin promotes rapid dynamic changes in hippocampal dendritic morphology." *Mol Cell Neurosci* 2007; 35(4):559–72.

Orwoll, E, et al. "Transdermal testosterone supplementation in normal older men." Paper presented at the annual meeting for the Endocrine Society, San Antonio, TX, June 24–27, 1992.

Oudshoorn, C, et al. "Higher serum vitamin D3 levels are associated with better cognitive test performance in patients with Alzheimer's disease." *Dement Geriatr Cogn Disord* 2008; 25(6): 539–43.

Paganini-Hill, A. "Alzheimer's disease in women." *The Female Patient* 1998, 23(3):10–20.

—. "Does estrogen replacement therapy protect against Alzheimer's disease?" *Osteoporosis Int* 1997; Supp 1:S12–17.

Paganini-Hill, A, and V Henderson. "Estrogen deficiency and risk of Alzheimer's disease in women." *Am J Epidemiology* 1994; 140(3):256–61.

—. "Estrogen replacement therapy and risk of Alzheimer's disease." *Arch Intern Med* 1996; 156(19):2213–7.

Peila, R, et al. "Fasting insulin and incident dementia: in an elderly population of Japanese-American men." *Neurology* 2004; 63(2):228–33.

—. "Type 2 diabetes APOE gene, and the risk for dementia and related pathologies: the Honolulu-Asia Aging Study." *Diabetes* 2002; 51(4):1256–62.

Perry, H, et al. "Longitudinal changes in serum 25-hydroxyvitamin D in older people." *Metabolism* 1999; 48(8):1028–32.

Phillips, S, and B Sherwin. "Effects of estrogen on memory function in surgically menopausal women." *Psychoneuroendocrinology* 1992; 17(5): 485–95.

Poehlman, E, et al. "Changes in energy balance and body composition at menopause: a controlled longitudinal study." *Ann Intern Med* 1995; 123(9):673–5.

Polcz, T, et al. "Effects of estrogen and progesterone on the central nervous system." In *Estrogens and Progestogens in Clinical Practice*, edited by I Fraser et al, 195–204. New York: Churchill Livingstone, 2000.

Power, D, et al., "Circulating leptin levels and weight loss in Alzheimer's disease patients." *Dement Geriatr Cogn Disord* 2001; 12(2):167–70.

Przybelski, R, and N Binkley. "Is vitamin D important for preserving cognition? A positive correlation of serum 25-hydroxyvitamin D concentration with cognitive function." *Arch Biochem Biophys* 2007; 460(2):202–5.

Przybelski, R, et al. "Rapid correction of low vitamin D status in nursing home residents." *Osteoporosis Int* 2008; 19(11):1621–8.

Puder, J, et al. "Estrogen modulates the hypothalamic-pituitary-adrenal and inflammatory cytokine responses to endotoxin in women." *J Clin Endocrinol Metab* 2001; 86(6):2403–8.

Rivas, M, et al. "Thyroid hormones, learning and memory." *Genes Brain Behav* 2007; 6 (Suppl 1):40–4.

Rocca, W, et al. "Increased risk of cognitive impairment of dementia in women who underwent oophorectomy before menopause." *Neurology* 2007; 69(11):1074–83.

Rosano, G, et al. "Acute anti-ischemic effect of testosterone in men with coronary artery disease." *Circulation* 1999; 99(13):1666–70.

Rosenthal, M, et al. "Hospitalization and mortality of diabetes in older adults. A 3-year prospective study." *Diabetes Care* 1998; 21(2):231–5.

Saad, F, and L Gooren. "The role of testosterone in the metabolic syndrome: a review." *J Steroid Biochem Mol Biol* 2009; 114(1–2):40–3.

Saad, F, et al. "The role of testosterone in the etiology and treatment of obesity, the metabolic syndrome, and diabetes mellitus type 2." *J Obes* 2011; 683–5.

Santisteban, P, and J Bernal. "Thyroid development and effect on the nervous system." *Rev Endocr Metab Disord* 2005; 6(3):217–28.

Sapolsky, R. "Why stress is bad for your brain." *Science* 1995; 273(5276):749–50.

Sarkar, N. "Hormonal profiles behind the heart of man." *Cardiol J* 2009; 16(4):300–6.

Schnaider Beeri, M, et al. "Diabetes mellitus in midlife and the risk of dementia three decades later." *Neurology* 2004; 63(10):1902–7.

Schumacher, M, et al. "Local synthesis and dual actions of progesterone in the nervous system: neuroprotection and myelination." *Growth Horm IGF Res* 2004; (Suppl A): S18–33.

Seamans, K, et al. "Vitamin D status and measures of cognitive function in healthy older European adults." *Eur J Clin Nutr* 2010; 64(10): 1172–8.

Selhub, E. "Stress and distress in clinical practice: a mind-body approach." *Nutr Clin Care* 2002; 5(4):182–90.

Shaywitz, S, et al. "Effect of estrogen on brain activation patterns in postmenopausal women during working memory tasks." *JAMA* 1999; 281(13): 1197–202.

Shors, T, et al. "Neurogenesis may relate to some but not all types of hippocampal-dependent learning." *Hippocampus* 2002; 12(5):578–84.

Simpkins, J, et al. "The potential for estrogens in preventing Alzheimer's disease and vascular dementia." *Adv Neurol Disord* 2009; 2(1):31–49.

—. "Role of estrogen replacement therapy in memory enhancement and the prevention of neuronal loss associated with Alzheimer's disease." *Am J Med* 1997; 103(3A):19S-25S.

Smith, J, et al. "Thyroid hormones, brain function, and cognition: a brief review." *Neurosci Biobehav Rev* 2002; 26(1):45–60.

Smith, P. *HRT: The Answers*. Traverse City, MI: Healthy Living Books, 2003.

—. *What You Must Know About Women's Hormones*. Garden City Park, NY: Square One Publishers, 2010.

Srinivasan, V, et al. "Melatonin and its agonist ramelteon in Alzheimer's disease: possible therapeutic value." *Int J Alzheimer's Dis* 2010.

Srivastava, R, et al. "Apolipoprotein E gene expression in various tissues of mouse and regulation by estrogen." *Biochem Mol Biol Int* 1996; 38(1):91–101.

Stangl, B, et al. "Administration of dehydroepiandrosterone (DHEA) enhances visual-spatial performance in postmenopausal women." *Behav Neurosci* 2011; 125(5):742–52.

Steen, E, et al. "Impaired insulin and insulin-like growth factor expression and signaling mechanisms in Alzheimer's disease—is this type-3 diabetes?" *J Alzheimer's Dis* 2005; 7(1):63–80.

Stevens, M, et al. "Low-dose estradiol alters brain activity." *Psychiatry Res* 2005; 139(3): 199–217.

Stuss, D, and Knight, R, editors. *Principles of Frontal Lobe Function*. New York: Oxford University Press, 2002.

Swanwick, G, et al. "Hypothalamic-pituitary-adrenal axis dysfunction in Alzheimer's disease: lack of association between longitudinal and cross-sectional findings." *Am J Psychiatry* 1998; 155(2):286–9.

Swerdloff, R, et al. "Androgen deficiency and aging in men." *West J Med* 1993; 159(5):579–85.

Tang, M, et al. "Effect of oestrogen during menopause on risk and age at onset of Alzheimer's disease." *Lancet* 1996; 348(9025): 429–32.

Tchernof, A, et al. "Sex steroid hormones, sex hormone-binding globulin, and obesity in men and women." *Horm Metab Res* 2000; 32(11–12): 526–36.

Tezapsidis, N, et al. "Leptin: a novel therapeutic strategy for Alzheimer's disease." *J Alzheimer's Dis* 2009; 16(4):731–40.

Thilers, P, et al. "The association between endogenous free testosterone and cognitive performance: a population based study in 35 to 90 year-old men and women." *Psychoneuroendocrinology* 2006; 31(5):565–76.

Tilvis, R, et al. "Predictors of cognitive decline and mortality of aged people over a 10-year period." *J Gerontol A Biol Sci Med Sci 2004*; 59(3):M268–74.

Tong, M, et al. "Mechanisms of ceramide-mediated neurodegeneration." *J Alz Dis* 2009; 16(4): 705–14.

Toran-Allerand, C, et al. "Estrogen receptors

colocalize with low affinity nerve growth factor receptors in cholinergic neurons of the basal forebrain." *Proc Natl Acad Sci* 1992; 89(10): 4668–72.

Tsolaki, M, et al. "Severe psychological stress in elderly individuals: a proposed model of neurodegeneration and its implications." *Am J Alzheimers Dis Other Demen* 2009; 24(2):85–94.

Tsuno, N, and A Homma. "What is the association between depression and Alzheimer's disease?" *Expert Rev Neurother* 2009; 9(11):1667–76.

Van den Beld, A, et al. "Measures of bioavailable serum testosterone and estradiol and their relationships with muscle strength, bone density, and body composition in elderly men." *J Clin Endocrinol Metab* 2000; 85(9):3276–82.

Van der Wielen, R, et al. "Serum vitamin D concentrations among elderly people in Europe." *Lancet* 1995; 346(8969):207–10.

Vasudevan, N, and D Pfaff. "Membrane-initiated actions of estrogens in neuroendocrinology: emerging principles." *Endocr Rev* 2007; 28(1):1–19.

Vermeulen, A. "Androgens in the aging male." *J Clin Endocrin Metab* 1991; 73(2):221–4.

Virtanen, M., et al. "Long working hours and cognitive function: The Whitehall II Study." *Am J Epidemiol* 2009; 169(5):596–605.

Wang, C, et al. "Investigation, treatment, and monitoring of late-onset hypogonadism in males: ISA, ISSAM, EAU, EAA, and ASA recommendations." *Eur J Endocrinol* 2008; 159(5): 507–14.

Warga, C. *Menopause and the Mind.* New York: Touchstone, 2000.

Watson, G, and S Craft. "The role of insulin resistance in the pathogenesis of Alzheimer's disease: implications for treatment." *CNS Drugs* 2003; 17(1):27–45.

Whipple, M, et al. "Hopelessness, depressive symptoms, and carotid atherosclerosis in women: The Study of Women's Health Across the Nation (SWAN) Heart Study." *Stroke* 2009; 40(10):3166–72.

White, Z. "Do you know your sex hormone status?" *Life Extension* May 2011, 30–6.

Wilcoxon, J, et al. "Behavioral inhibition and impaired spatial learning and memory in hypothyroid mice lacking thyroid hormone receptor alpha." *Behav Brain Res* 2007; 177(1):109–116.

Wilkins, C, et al. "Vitamin D deficiency is associated with low mood and worse cognitive performance in older adults." *Am J Geriatr Psychiatry* 2006; 14(12):1032–40.

Williams, G, and P Goldman-Rakic. "Modulation of memory fields by dopamine D1 receptors in prefrontal cortex." *Nature* 1995; 376(6541):572–5.

Wilson, R, et al. "Chronic distress, age-related neuropathology, and late-life dementia." *Psychosom Med* 2007; 69(1):47–53.

Wise, P, et al. "Minireview: neuroprotective effects of estrogen—new insights into mechanisms of action." *Endocrinology* 2001; 142(3): 969–73.

Wong, M, and R Moss. "Long-term and short-term electrophysiological effects of estrogen on the synaptic properties of hippocampal CA1 neurons." *J Neuroscience* 1992; 12(8):3217–25.

Yaffe, K, et al. "Apolipoprotein E phenotype and cognitive decline in a prospective study of elderly community women." *Arch Neurol* 1998; 54(9):1110–4.

—. "Sex hormones and cognitive function in older men." *J Am Geriatr Soc* 2002; 50(4):707–12.

—. "Estrogen therapy in postmenopausal women: effects on cognitive function and dementia." *JAMA* 1998; 279(9):688–95.

Yeap, B. "Testosterone and ill-health in aging men." *Nat Clin Pract Endocrinol Metab* 2009; 5(2):113–21.

Zandi, P, et al. "Hormone replacement therapy and incidence of Alzheimer's disease in older women." *JAMA* 2002; 288(17):2123–9.

Chapter 5: Inflammation

Agarwal, K. "Therapeutic actions of garlic constitutents." *Med Res Rev* 1996; 16(1):111–124.

Appleton, N. *Lick The Sugar Habit.* Garden City Park, New York: Avery Publishing Group, 1995.

—. *Stopping Inflammation: Relieving the Cause of Degenerative Diseases.* Garden City Park, NY: Square One Publishers, 2005.

Avramoglu, R, et al. "Mechanisms of metabolic dyslipidemia in insulin resistant states: deregulation of hepatic and intestinal lipoprotein secretion." *Front Biosci* 2003; 8:464–76.

Aziz, N, et al. "Comparative antibacterial and

antifungal effects of some phenolic compounds." *Microbios* 1998; 93(374):43–54.

Basciano, H, et al. "Fructose, insulin resistance, and metabolic dyslipidemia." *Nutr Metab:* 2005: 2(1):5.

Beck-Nielsen, H, et al. "Effects of diet on the cellular insulin binding and the insulin sensitivity in young healthy subjects." *Diabetologia* 1978; 15(4):289–96.

—. "Impaired cellular insulin binding and insulin sensitivity induced by high-fructose feeding in normal subjects." *Am J Clin Nutr* 1980; 33(2):273–8.

Beloin, N, et al. "Ethnomedicinal uses of momordicaharantia (Cucurbitaceae) in Togo and relation to its phytochemistry and biological activity." *J Ethnopharmacol* 2005; 96(1–2):49–55.

Berkson, D. *Healthy Digestion the Natural Way.* New York: John Wiley & Sons, 2000.

Bland, J, et al, editors. *Clinical Nutrition: A Functional Approach.* Gig Harbor, WA: The Institute for Functional Medicine, 1999.

Blum, S, et al. "Effect of a Mediterranean meal on postprandial carotenoids, paraoxonase and C-reactive protein levels." *Ann Nutr Metabol* 2006; 50(1):20–4.

Blumenthal, M, editor. *The Complete German Commission E Monographs: Therapeutic Guide to Herbal Medicines.* Boston: American Botanical Council, 1998.

Bronwell, L. "What doctors don't know about inflammation." *Life Extension,* January 2013, 39–47.

Bruunsgaard, H. "Physical activity and modulation of systemic low-level inflammation." *J Leukoc Biol* 2005; 78(4):819–35.

Bunn, F, et al. "Reaction of monosaccharides with protein possible evolutionary significance." *Science* 1981; 213(4504):222–4.

Burrascano, J. *Advanced Topics in Lyme Disease: Diagnostic Hints and Treatment Guidelines for Lyme and Other Tick Borne Illnesses.* East Hampton, NY: East End Medical Associates, 2000.

Calliste, C, et al. "Free radical scavenging activities measured by electron spin resonance spectroscopy and B16 cell antiproliferative behaviors of seven plants." *J Agric Food Chem* 2001; 49(7):3321–7.

Cameron, D, et al. "Evidence –based guidelines for the management of Lyme disease," *Expert Rev Anti Infect Ther* 2004; 2(Suppl 1):S1–S13.

Cassarino, D, et al. "Lyme-associated parkinsonism: a neuropathologic case study and review of the literature." *Arch Pathol Lab Med* 2003; 127(9):1204–6.

Cerami, A, et al. "Glucose and aging." *Sci Am* 1987; 256(5):90–6.

Challem, J. *The Inflammation Syndrome.* Hoboken, NJ: John Wiley & Sons, 2003.

Chin, R, and N Latov. "Peripheral neuropathy and celiac disease." *Curr Treat Options Neurol* 2005; 7(1):43–8.

Chin, R, et al. "Neurologic complications of celiac disease." *J Clin Neuromusc Dis* 2004; 5(3): 129–37.

Chung, H, et al. "Molecular inflammation: underpinnings of aging and age-related disease." *Ageing Res Rev* 2009; 8(1):18–30.

Colgan, M. *The New Nutrition.* Vancouver, BC, Canada: Apple Tree Publishing, 1996.

Comalada, M, et al. "In vivo quercitrin anti-inflammatory effect involves release of quercetin, which inhibits inflammation through down-regulation of the NF-kappa B pathway." *Eur J Immunol* 2005; 35(2):584–92.

Cook, W. *The Yeast Connection Handbook.* Garden City Park, NY: Square One Publishers, 2007.

Coulter, P, et al. "Two-year evaluation of Borrelia burgdorferi culture and supplemental tests for definitive diagnosis of Lyme disease." *J Clin Microbiol* 2005; 43(10):5080–84.

Cvetnic, Z, and S Vladimir-Knezevic. "Antimicrobial activity of grapefruit seed and pulp ethanolic extract." *Acta Pharm* 2004; 54(3): 243–50.

Darlington, L, et al. "Placebo-controlled, blind study of dietary manipulation therapy in rheumatoid arthritis." *Lancet* 1986; 8475(1): 236–8.

Dattwyler, R, et al. "Treatment of late Lyme borreliosis—randomized comparison of ceftriaxone and penicillin." *Lancet* 1988; 1(8596):1191–4.

Dickey, W. "Epilepsy, cerebral calcifications, and celiac disease." *Lancet* 1994; 344(8937):1585–6.

Dietrich, M, and I Jialal. "The effect of weight loss on a stable biomarker of inflammation, C-reactive protein." *Nutr Rev* 2005; 63(1):22–8.

Dyer, D, et al. "Accumulation of maillard reaction products in skin collagen in diabetes and aging." *J Clin Invest* 1993; 91(6):2463–9.

Elliott, S, et al. "Fructose, weight gain, and the insulin resistance syndrome." *Am J Clin Nutr* 2002; 76(5):911–22.

Erasmus, Udo. *Fats That Heal, Fats That Kill.* Burnaby, BC, Canada: Alive Books, 1993.

Fallon, B, et al. "Late-stage neuropsychiatric Lyme borreliosis. Differential diagnosis and treatment." *Psychosomatics* 1995; 36(3):295–300.

—. "A randomized, placebo-controlled trial of repeated IV antibiotic therapy for Lyme encephalopathy." *Neurology* 2008; 70(13):992–1003.

Fasano, A, and C Catassi. "Current approaches to diagnosis and treatment of celiac disease: an evolving spectrum." *Gastroenterol* 2001; 120(3):636–51.

Feder, H, et al. "A critical appraisal of 'chronic Lyme disease.'" *NEJM* 2007; 357(14):1422–30.

Flavin, D. "Metabolic danger of high-frutose corn syrup." *Life Extension,* Dec 2008, 69–77.

Franceschi, C. "Inflammaging a major characteristic of old people: can it be prevented or cured?" *Nutr Rev* 2007; 65(12 Pt 2):S173–6.

Galland, L. "Intestinal protozoan infestation and systemic illness." In *Textbook of Natural Medicine,* edited by J Pizzorno and M Murray. St. Louis, MO: Elsevier, 2006, p. 655–9.

Gasser, R, et al. "Reversal of Borrelia burgdorferi associated dilated cardiomyopathy by antibiotic: treatment?" *Cardiovasc Drugs Ther* 1996; 10(3):351–60.

Giove, R. "Traditional medicine in the treatment of enteroparasitosis." *Rev Gastroenterol Peru* 1996; 16(3):197–202.

Gitler, C, et al., "Factors contributing to the pathogenic behavior of Entamoeba histolytica," *Ann Rev Microbiol* 1986; 40:237–61.

Glinsmann, W, et al. "Report from FDA's Sugar Task Force, 1986: evaluation of health aspects of sugars contained in carbohydrate sweeteners." *J Nutr* 1986; 116(Suppl 1).

Golightly, M, et al. "ELISA and immunoblots in the diagnosis of Lyme borreliosis: sensitivities and sources of false-positive results." In *Lyme Disease: Molecular and Immunologic Approaches,* edited by S Schutzer, 283–298. Plainview, NY: Cold Spring Harbor Laboratory Press, 1992.

—. "The laboratory diagnosis of Lyme borreliosis." *Lab Med* 1990; 21:299–304.

Goodman, J. *The Omega Solution.* Roseville, CA: Prima Publishing, 2001.

Graham, D, et al. "Why do apparently healthy people use antacid tablets?" *Am J Gastroenterol* 1983; 78(5):257–60.

Green, P. *Celiac Disease.* New York: William Morrow, 2010.

Green, P, and B Jabri. "Celiac disease." *Lancet* 2003; 362(9381):383–91.

Green, P, et al. "Risk of malignancy in patients with celiac disease." *Am J Med* 2003; 115(3): 191–5.

Greenberg, A, and M Obin. "Obesity and the role of adipose tissue in inflammation and metabolism." *Am J Clin Nutr* 2006; 83(2):461S–5S.

Gross, L, et al. "Increased consumption of refined carbohydrates and the epidemic of type 2 diabetes in the United States: an ecologic assessment." *Am J Clin Nutr* 2004; 79(5):774–9.

Gruenwald, J, et al. *PDR for Herbal Medicine.* First Edition. Montvale, NJ: Medical Economics Company, 1998.

Guilliams, T. "Managing chronic inflammation: natural solutions." *The Standard* 2006; 7(2):1–8.

Gupte, S. "Use of berberine in treatment of giardiasis." *Am J Dis Child* 1975; 129(7):866.

Halperin, J, et al. "Lyme disease: cause of a treatable peripheral neuropathy." *Neurology* 1987; 37(11):1700–6.

—. "Practice parameter: treatment of nervous system Lyme disease (an evidence-based review): Report of the Quality Standards Subcommittee of the American Academy of Neurology." *Neurology* 2007; 69(1):91–102.

Hammond, R, et al. "Alzheimer's disease and spirochetes: a questionable relationship" *Neuroreport* 1993; 4(7):840.

Hien, T, et al. "Qinghaosu." *Lancet* 1993; 341(8845):603–8.

Hiscock, N, et al. "Glutamine supplementation further enhances exercise-induced plasma IL-6." *J Appl Physiol* 2003; 95(1):145–48.

Hwang, B, et al. "Antimicrobial constituents from goldenseal (the Rhizomes of Hydratis canadensis) against selected oral pathogens." *Planta Medica* 2003; 69(7):623–7.

Jenny, N, et al. "Long-term assessment of inflammation and healthy aging in late life: The Cardiovascular Health Study All Stars." *J Gerontol A Biol Sci Med Sci* 2012; 67(9):970–6.

Kalemba, D, and A Kunicka. "Antibacterial and antifungal properties of essential oils." *Curr Med Chem* 2003; 10(10):813–29.

Kang, O, et al. "Inhibition of interleukin-8 production in the human colonic epithelial cell line HT-29 by 18 beta-glycyrrhetinic acid," *Int J Mol Med* 2005; 15(6):981–85.

Keen, H, et al. "Nutrient intake, adiposity, and diabetes." *Br Med J* 1979; 6164(1):655–8.

Klempner, M, et al. "Two controlled trials of antibiotic treatment in patients with persistent symptoms and a history of Lyme disease." *NEJM* 2001; 345(2):85–92.

Kohler, J. "Lyme borreliosis in neurology and psychiatry." *Fortschr Med* 1990; 108(10):191–3, 197.

Kruis, W, et al. "Effects of diets low and high in refined sugars on gut transit, bile acid metabolism, and bacterial fermentation." *Gut* 1991; 32(4):367–71.

Lee, A, and A Cerami. "Modifications of proteins and nucleic acids by reducing sugars: possible role in aging." In *Handbook of the Biology of Aging*, edited by Edward Schneider, 116–30. San Diego, CA: Academic Press, 1990.

Lemann, J, et al. "Evidence that glucose ingestion inhibits net renal tubular reabsorption of calcium and magnesium in man." *J Lab Clin Med* 1970; 75(4):578–85.

Lerman, R. "The essential fatty acids in psychiatric and neurological dysfunction." *Brain Biochemistry and Nutrition*. Gig Harbor, WA: The Institute for Functional Medicine, 2002.

—. "Nutrients as biological response modifiers: fatty acids and inflammation." *Applying Functional Medicine in Clinical Practice*. Gig Harbor,

WA: The Institute for Functional Medicine, 2002.

Liu, S, et al. "Relation between a diet with a high glycemic load and plasma concentrations of high-sensitivity C-reactive protein in middle-aged women." *Am J Clin Nutr* 2002; 75(3):492–8.

Logigian, E. "Peripheral nervous system Lyme borreliosis." *Semin Neurol* 1997; 17(1):25–30.

Ma, B, et al. "Serodiagnosis of Lyme borreliosis by western immunoblot: reactivity of various significant antibodies against Borrelia burgdorferi." *J Clin Microbiol* 1992; 30(2):370–76.

Macdonald, S, and P Bennett. *Textbook of Functional Medicine*. Gig Harbor WA: Institute for Functional Medicine, 2006.

McLain, N, et al. "Undecylenic acid inhibits morphogenesis of Candida albicans." *Antimicrob Agents Chemother* 2000; 44(10):2873–5.

Miklossy, J. "Alzheimer's disease—a spirochetosis?" *Neuroreport* 1993; 4(7):841–8.

Miller, G, et al. "Chronic psychological stress and the regulation of pro-inflammatory cytokines: a glucocorticoid-resistance model." *Health Psychol* 2002; 21(6): 531–41.

Morley, J. "The aging gut: physiology." *Clin Geriatr Med* 2007; 23(4):757–67.

Murray, J, et al. "Trends in the identification and clinical features of celiac disease in a North American community: 1950–2001." *Clin Gastroenterol Hepatol* 2003; 1(1):19–27.

Nicklas, B, et al. "Behavioral treatments for chronic systemic inflammation: effects of dietary weight loss and exercise training." *CMAJ* 2005; 72(9):1199–209.

Otamiri, T, and C Tagesson. "Ginkgo biloba extract prevents mucosal damage associated with small-intestinal ischemia." *Scand J Gastroenterol* 1989; 24(6):666–70.

Pachner, A. "Neurologic manifestations of Lyme disease, the new 'great imitator.'" *Rev Infect Dis* 1989; 11(Suppl 6):51482–6.

—. "The triad of neurologic manifestations of Lyme disease: meningitis, cranial neuritis, and radioculoneuritis." *Neurology* 1985; 35(1):47–53.

Pachner, A, et al. "Central nervous system manifestations of Lyme disease." *Arch Neurol* 1989; 46(7):790–5.

Park, S, et al. "Preventive effect of the flavonoid, wogonin, against ethanol-induced gastric mucosal damage in rats." *Dig Dis Sci* 2004; 49(3): 384–94.

Persson, B, et al. "Diet and inflammatory bowel disease." *Epidemiology* 1992; 3(1):47–52.

Pfister, H, et al. "Catatonic syndrome in acute severe encephalitis due to Borrelia burgdorferi infection." *Neurology* 1993; 43(2):433–5.

Pieroni, A, et al. "In vitro anti-complementary activity of flavonoids from olive (Olea europaea L.) leaves." *Pharmazie* 1996; 51(10):765–8.

Pischon, T, et al. "Habitual dietary intake of n-3 and n-6 fatty acids in relation to inflammatory markers among US men and women." *Circulation* 2003; 108(2):155–160.

Ponikau, J, et al. "The diagnosis and incidence of allergic fungal sinusitis." *Mayo Clinic Proceedings* 1999; 74(9):877–84.

Qi, L, et al. "Whole-grain, bran, and cereal fiber intakes and markers of systemic inflammation in diabetic women." *Diabetes Care* 2006; 29(2): 207–11.

Quillin, P. *Beating Cancer With Nutrition.* Tulsa, Oklahoma: Nutrition Times Press, 2001.

Rakel, D, and A Rindfleisch. "Inflammation: nutritional, botanical, and mind-body influences." *South Med J* 2005; 98(3):303–10.

Reik, L, et al. "Demyelinating encephalopathy in Lyme disease." *Neurology* 1985; 35(2):267–69.

—. "Neurologic abnormalities of Lyme disease." *Medicine* 1979; 58(4):281–94.

Reiser, S, et al. "Effect of dietary sugars on metabolic risk factors associated with heart disease." *Nutr Health* 1985; 3(4):203–16.

Ringsdorf, W, et al. "Sucrose neutrophilic phagocytosis and resistance to disease." *Dent Surv* 1976; 52(12):46–8.

Romi, F, et al. "Neuroborreliosis and vasculitis causing stroke-like manifestations," *Eur Neurol* 2004; 51(1):49–50.

Rountree, R. "Immune dysfunction and inflammation, Part II." *Applying Functional Medicine in Clinical Practice.* Gig Harbor, WA: The Institute for Functional Medicine, 2002.

Sakai, H, and M Misawa. "Effect of sodium azulene sulfonate on capsaicin-induced pharyngitis in rats." Basic Clin Pharmacol Toxicol 2005; 96(1):54–9.

Sanchez, A, et al. "Role of sugars in human neutrophilic phagocytosis." *AmJ Clin Nutr* 1973; 26(11):1180–4.

Sander, H, et al. "Cerebralar ataxia and celiac disease." *Lancet* 2003; 362(9395):1548.

Schmidt, M. *Brain-Building Nutrition: The Healing Power of Fats and Oils.* Berkeley, CA: Frog Books, 2006.

Sierra, S, et al. "IL-10 expression is involved in the regulation of the immune response by omega-3 fatty acids." *Nutr Hosp* 2004; 19(6): 376–82.

Sies, H, et al. "Nutritional, dietary, and postprandial oxidative stress." *J Nutr* 2005; 135(5): 969–72.

Sivak, S, et al. "Accuracy of IgM immunoblotting to confirm the clinical diagnosis of early Lyme disease." *Arch Int Med* 1996; 156(18): 2105–09.

Smith, P. *Vitamins: Hype or Hope?* Traverse City, MI: Healthy Living Books, 2004.

Subbaiah, T, and A Amin. "Effect of berberine sulphate on Entamoeba histolytica." *Nature* 1967; 215:527–8.

Vanderhoof-Forschner, K. *Everything You Need To Know About Lyme Disease and Other Tick-Borne Disorders.* Hoboken, NJ: John Wiley & Sons, Inc., 2003.

Ventura, A, et al. "Duration of exposure to gluten and risk for autoimmune disorders in patients with celiac disease." *Gastroenterol* 1999; 117(2):297–303.

Vos, M, et al. "Dietary fructose consumption among U.S. children and adults: The Third National Health and Nutrition Examination Survey." *Medscape J Med* 2008; 10(7):160.

Waisbren, B, et al. "Borrelia burgdorferi antibodies and amyotrophic lateral sclerosis." *Lancet* 1987; 2(8554):332–3.

Wang, H, and T Ng. "Isolation of cucurmoschin, a novel antifungal peptide abundant in arginine, glutamate, and glycine residues from black pumpkin seeds." *Peptides* 2003; 24(7):969–72.

Weintraub, P. *Cure Unknown: Inside The Lyme Epidemic*. New York: St. Martin's Press, 2009.

Welbourne, T, et al. "An oral glutamine load enhances renal acid secretion and function." *Am J Clin Nutr* 1998; 67(4):660–63.

Wittner, M, and R Rosenbaum. "Role of bacteria in modifying virulence of E. histolytica: studies of amoebae from axenic cultures," *Am J Trop Med Hyg* 1970; 19(5):755–61.

Chapter 6: Insomnia

Altun, A, and B Uqur-Altun. "Melatonin: therapeutic and clinical utilization." *Int J Clin Pract* 2007; 61(5):835–45.

Armstrong, D. *Herbs That Work: The Scientific Evidence of Their Healing Powers*. Berkeley, CA: Ulysses Press, 2001.

Autret, A, et al. "Human sleep and 5-HTP: effects of repeated high doses and of association with benserazide." *Electroencephalogr Clin Neurophysiol* 1976; 41(4):408–13.

Birdsall, T. "5-hydroxytryptophan: a clinically-effective serotonin precursor." *Altern Med Rev* 1998; 3(4):271–80.

Boon, H, and M Smith. *Complete Natural Medicine Guide to the 50 Most Common Medicinal Herbs*. Toronto: Robert Rose, 2004.

Born, J, et al. "Effects of sleep and circadian rhythm on human circulating immune cells." *J Immunol* 1997; 158(9):4454–64.

Brzezinski, A, et al. "Effects of exogenous melatonin on sleep: a meta-analysis." *Sleep Med Rev* 2005; 9(1):41–50.

Brown, S, et al. "Occult caffeine as a source of sleep problems in an older population." *J Am Geriatr Soc* 1995; 43(8):860–4.

Burgos, I, et al. "Increased nocturnal interleukin-6 excretion in patients with primary insomnia: a pilot study." *Brain Behav Immun* 2006; 20(3):246–53.

Gaby, A. *Nutritional Medicine*. Concord, NH: Fritz Perlberg Publishing, 2011.

George, C, et al. "The effect of L-tryptophan on daytime sleep latency in normals: correlation with blood levels." *Sleep* 1989; 12(4):345–53.

Gerstner, J, and J Yin. "Circadian rhythms and memory formation." *Nat Rev Neurosci* 2010; 11(8):577–88.

Greden, J. "Anxiety or caffeinism: a diagnostic dilemma." *Am J Psychiatry* 1974; 131(10): 1089–92.

Gutierrez, S, et al. "Assessing subjective and psychomotor effects of the herbal medication valerian in healthy volunteers." *Pharmacol Biochem Behav* 2004; 78(1):57–64.

Hadley, S. "Valerian." *Am Fam Physician* 2003; 67(8):1755–8.

Hallam, K, et al. "Comparative cognitive and psychomotor effects of single doses of Valeriana officinalis and triazolam in healthy volunteers." *Hum Psychopharmacol* 2003; 18(8):619–25.

Hardy, M, et al. "Replacement of drug treatment for insomnia by ambient odor." *Lancet* 1995; 346(8976):701.

Hartmann, E. "L-tryptophan: a rational hypnotic with clinical potential." *Am J Psychiatry* 1977; 134(4):366–70.

Hastings, M, et al. "A clockwork web: circadian timing in brain and periphery, in health and disease." *Nat Rev Neurosci* 2003; 4(8):649–61.

Herzog, E. "Neurons and networks in daily rhythms." *Nat Rev Neurosci* 2007; 8(10):790–802.

Irwin, M, et al. "Sleep deprivation and activation of morning levels of cellular and genomic markers of inflammation." *Arch Intern Med* 2006; 166(16):1756–62.

Kapsimalis, F, et al. "Cytokines and pathological sleep." *Sleep Med* 2008, 9(6):603–14.

Klatz, R, and R Goldman. *The New Anti-Aging Revolution*. North Bergen, NJ: Basic Health Publications, 2003.

Landolt, H, et al. "Late-afternoon ethanol intake affects nocturnal sleep and sleep EEG in middle-aged men." *J Clin Psychopharmacol* 1996; 16(6):428–36.

Larzelere, M, et al. "Anxiety, depression, and insomnia." *Prim Care* 2002; 29(2):339–60.

Leathwood, P, et al. "Quantifying the effects of mild sedatives." *J Psychiatr Res* 1982; 17(2): 115–22.

Leprout, R, et al. "Sleep loss results in elevation of cortisol levels the next evening." *Sleep* 1997; 20(10):865–70.

Lynch, H, et al. "Daily rhythm in human urinary melatonin." *Science* 1975; 187(4172):169–71.

Mayo Clinic. "Insomnia." Last modified January 7, 2011. www.mayoclinic.com/health/insomnia/DS00187.

Meier-Ewert H, et al. "Effect of sleep loss on C-reactive protein, an inflammatory marker of cardiovascular risk." *J Am Coll Cardiol* 2004; 43(4):678–83.

Morin, C, et al. "Valerian-hops combination and diphenhydramine for treating insomnia: a randomized placebo-controlled clinical trial." *Sleep* 2005; 28(11):1465–71.

Murray, M, "Insomnia." In *Textbook of Natural Medicine*, edited by J Pizzorno and M Murray, 1552–6. St. Louis, MO: Elsevier, 2013.

Naiman, R. "Insomnia." In *Integrative Medicine*, edited by D Rakel, 65–76. Philadelphia: Elsevier/Saunders, 2013.

National Heart, Lung, and Blood Institute. "What Causes Insomnia?" Last modified December 13, 2011. www.nhlbi.nih.gov/health/health-topics/topics/inso/causes.html.

Nave, R, et al. "Melatonin improves evening napping." *Eur J Pharmacol* 1995; 275(2):213–6.

Pace-Schott, E, and J Hobson. "The neurobiology of sleep: genetics, cellular physiology and subcortical networks." *Nat Neurosci Rev* 2002; 3(8):591–605.

Roberts, H. "Reactions attributed to aspartame-containing products: 551 cases." *J Appl Nutr* 1988; 40(8):5–94.

Robinson, C, et al. "The effects of nicotinamide upon sleep in humans" *Biol Psychiatry* 1977; 12(1):139–43.

Roth, T, and T Roehrs. "Insomnia: epidemiology, characteristics, and consequences." *Clin Cornerstone* 2003; 5(3):5–15.

Rowe, A. "Perennial nasal allergy due to food sensitization." *J Asthma Res* 1966; 3(2):141–54.

Smidt, L, et al. "Influence of thiamin supplementation on the health and general well-being of an elderly Irish population with marginal thiamin deficiency." *J Gerontol* 1991; 46(1):M16–22.

Smith, P. *What You Must Know About Vitamins, Minerals, Herbs, and More*. Garden City Park, NY: Square One Publishers, 2008.

Stevenson, C, and E Ernst. "Valerian for insomnia: a systematic review of randomized clinical trials." *Sleep Med* 2000; 1(2):91–9.

Tiffin, P, et al. "Pharmacokinetic and pharmacodynamics responses to caffeine in poor and normal sleepers." *Psychopharmacology* 1995; 121(4):494–502.

University of Maryland Medical Center. "Insomnia." Last modified June 25, 2013. http://umm.edu/health/medical/reports/articles/insomnia.

Vermeeren, A. "Residual effects of hypnotics: epidemiology and clinical implications." *CNS Drugs* 2004; 18(5):297–328.

Vitiello, M. "Sleep, alcohol, and alcohol abuse." *Addict Biol* 1997; 2(2):151–8.

Weiner, M. *Weiner's Herbal: The Guide to Herb Medicine*. Mill Valley, CA: Quantum Books, 1990.

Weiss, R, and V Fintelmann. *Herbal Medicine*. New York: Thierne, 2000.

Wilkinson, T, et al. "The response to treatment of subclinical thiamine deficiency in the elderly." *Am J Clin Nutr* 1997; 66(4):925–8.

Willner, C. "The importance of sleep in a functional medicine module." Paper presented at the Fellowship in Anti-Aging, Regenerative and Functional Medicine, November 1–3, 2012, Atlanta, GA.

Wyatt, R. "The serotonin-catecholamine-dream bicycle: a clinical study." *Biol Psychiatry* 1972; 5(1):133–64.

Wyatt, R, et al. "Effects of 5-hydroxytryptophan on the sleep of normal human subjects." *Electroencephalogr Clin Neurophysiol* 1971; 30(6):505–9.

Yamada, T, et al. "Effect of theanine, r-glutamylethylamide, on neurotransmitter release and its relationship with glutamic acid neurotransmission." *Nutr Neurosci* 2005; 8(4):219–26.

Zick, S, et al. "Preliminary examination of the efficacy and safety of a standardized chamomile extract for chronic primary insomnia: a randomized placebo-controlled pilot study." *BMC Complement Altern Med* 2001; 11:78.

Ziegler, G, et al. "Efficacy and tolerability of valerian extract L1 156 compared with oxazepam in the treatment of nonorganic insomnia: a randomized, double-blind, comparative clinical study." *Eur J Med Res* 2002; 7(11):480–6.

Chapter 7: Dementia

Aarsland, D, et al. "Memantine in patients with Parkinson's disease dementia or dementia with Lewy bodies: a double-blind, placebo-controlled multicenter trial." *Lancet Neurol* 2009; 8(7):613–8.

Alzheimer's Association. "What is Dementia?" Accessed August 28, 2013.www.alz.org/what-is-dementia.asp.Birks, J. "Cholinesterase inhibitors for Alzheimer's disease." *Cochrane Database Syst Rev* 2006; 25(1):CD005593.

Association for Frontotemporal Degeneration. "What is FTD?" Accessed August 29, 2013. www.theaftd.org/frontotemporal-degeneration.

Blennow, K, et al. "Tau protein in cerebrospinal fluid: a biochemical marker for axonal degeneration in Alzheimer disease?" *Mol Chem Neuropathol* 1995; 26(3):231–45.

Budson, A, and P Solomon. *Memory Loss: A Practical Guide for Clinicians*. Philadelphia: Elsevier/Saunders, 2011.

Bullock, R, et al. "Rivastigmine and donepezil treatment in moderate to moderately-severe Alzheimer's disease over a 2-year period." *Curr Med Res Opin* 2005; 21(8):1317–27.

Davis, K, et al. "Cholinergic markers in elderly patients with early signs of Alzheimer disease." *JAMA* 1999; 281(15):1401–6

House, E, et al. "Copper abolishes the B-sheet secondary structure of preformed amyloid fibrils of amyloid-B." *J Alzheimer's Dis* 2009; 18(4):811–7.

Hung, Y, et al. "Copper in the brain and Alzheimer's disease." *J Biol Inorg Chem* 2010; 15(1):61–76.

Jones, R, et al. "A multinational, randomized, 12-week study comparing the effects of donepezil and galantamine in patients with mild to moderate Alzheimer's disease." *Int J Geriatr Psychiatry* 2004; 19(1):58–67.

Lewy Body Dementia Association. "What is LBD?" Accessed August 29, 2013.www.lbda.org/category/3437/what-is-lbd.htm.

Lopez, O, et al. "Long-term effects of the concomitant use of memantine with cholinesterase inhibition in Alzheimer disease." *J Neurol Neurosurg Psychiatry* 2009; 80(6):600–7.

Markesbery, W. "Oxidative stress hypothesis in Alzhiemer's disease." *Free Radic Biol Med* 1997; 23(1):134–47.

Mayo Clinic. "Dementia," Last updated April 16, 2013. www.mayoclinic.com/health/dementia/DS01131.

National Institute of Neurological Disorders and Stroke. "Dementia: Hope Through Research," Last modified June 26, 2013. www.ninds.nih.gov/disorders/dementias/detail_dementia.htm#2300019213.

Perry, G, et al. "Alzheimer disease and oxidative stress." *J Biomed Biotechnol* 2002; 2(3): 120–3.

Plassman, B, et al. "Prevalence of dementia in the united states: the aging, demographics, and memory study." *Neuroepidemiology* 2007; 29(1–2):125–132.

Reisberg, B, et al. "Memantine in moderate-to-severe Alzheimer's disease," *NEJM* 2003; 348(14):1333–41.

Thies, W, et al. "2013 Alzheimer's Disease Facts and Figures." *Alzheimer's Dementia* 2013; 9(2): 208–45.

Walsh, W. *Nutrient Power: Heal Your Biochemistry and Heal Your Brain*. New York: Skyhorse Publishing, 2012.

Wilcock, G, et al. "A long-term comparison of galantamine and donepezil in the treatment of Alzhiemer's disease." *Drugs Aging* 2003; 20(10):777–89.

Yang, X, et al. "Coordinating to three histidine residues: Cu (II) promotes oligometric and fibrillar amyloid-B peptide to precipitate in a non-B-aggregation manner." *J Alzheimer's Dis* 2009; 18(4):799–810.

Zhang, Q, et al. "Metabolite-initiated protein misfolding may trigger Alzheimer's disease." *Proc Natl Acad Sci* 2004; 101(14):4752–7.

Chapter 8: Physical Activity

American College of Sports Medicine. "Reducing Sedentary Behaviors: Sitting Less and Moving More." Indianapolis, IN: ACSM, 2011.

Cassilhas, R, et al. "Spatial memory is improved by aerobic and resistance exercise through divergent molecular mechanisms." *Neuroscience* 2012; 202: 309–17.

Centers for Disease Control and Prevention. "Adult Participation in Aerobic and Muscle-Strengthening Physical Activities—United States, 2011." *MMWR Morb Mortal Wkly Rep* 2013; 62(17):326–30.

Chaouloff, F. "Physical exercise and brain monoamines: a review." *Acta Physiol Scand* 1989; 137(1): 1–13.

Cotman, C. "Synaptic plasticity, neurotrophic factors, and transplantation in the aged brain." in *Handbook of the Biology of Aging,* edited by E Schneider and J Rowe, 225–74. New York: Academic Press, 1990.

Cotman, C, and N Berchtold. "Exercise: a behavioral intervention to enhance brain health and plasticity." *Trends Neurosci* 2002; 25(6): 295–301.

Diamond, M, et al. "Differences in occipital cortical synapses from environmentally enriched, impoverished, and standard colony rats." *J Neurosci Res* 1975; 1(2):109–119.

Erickson, K, and A Kramer. "Aerobic exercise effects on cognitive and neural plasticity in older adults." *Br J Sports Med* 2009; 43: 22–24.

Erickson, K, et al. "Exercise training increases size of hippocampus and improves memory." *PNAS* 2011; 108(7): 3017–3022.

Garber, C, et al. "Quantity and quality of exercise for developing and maintaining cardiorespiratory, musculoskeletal, and neuromotor fitness in apparently healthy adult: guidance for prescribing exercise." *Med Sci Sports Exercise* 2011; 43(7):1334–59.

Goldman, R. *Brain Fitness.* New York: Doubleday, 1998.

Grimm, J. "Interaction of physical activity and diet: implications for insulin-glucose dynamics." *Public Health Nutr* 1999; 2(3A):363–8.

Hillman, C, et al. "Be smart, exercise your heart: exercise effects on brain and cognition." *Nat Rev Neurosci* 2008; 9(1):58–65.

Horber, F, et al. "Effect of regular physical training on age-associated alteration of body composition in men." *Eur J Clin Invest* 1996; 26(4):279–85.

Hughes, F, et al. "Exercise increases muscle

GLUT-4 levels and insulin action in subjects with impaired glucose tolerance." *Am J Physiol* 1993; 264(6):E855–62.

Jedrziewski, M, et al. "Exercise and cognition: results from the National Long Term Care Study." *Alzheimers Dement* 2010; 6(6):448–55.

Khalsa, D. "Alzheimer Disease." In *Integrative Medicine,* edited by D Rakel, 78–90. Philadelphia: Elsevier/Saunders, 2013.

Knaepen, K, et al. "Neuroplasticity: exercise-induced response of peripheral brain-derived neurotrophic factor: a systematic review of experimental studies in human subjects." *Sports Med* 2010; 40(9): 765–801.

Larson, E. "Physical activity for older adults at risk for Alzheimer disease." *JAMA* 2008; 300(9):1077–9.

Lee, I-Min, et al. "Effect of physical inactivity on major noncommunicable diseases worldwide: an analysis of burden of disease and life expectancy." *Lancet* 2012; 380(9839):219–29.

Lehmann, R, et al. "Loss of abdominal fat and improvement of the cardiovascular risk profile by regular moderate exercise training in patients with NIDDM." *Diabetologia* 1995; 38(11):1313–9.

Liu-Ambrose, T, et al. "Resistance training and executive functions in a 12-month randomized controlled trial." *Arch Intern Med* 2010; 170(2): 170–8.

Reynolds, G. "How exercise could lead to a better brain." *New York Times,* April 22, 2012, accessed September 16, 2013. www.nytimes.com/2012/04/22/magazine/how-exercise-could-lead-to-a-better-brain.html?pagewanted=all.

Rhodes, J, et al. "Exercise increases hippocampal neurogenesis to high levels but does not improve spatial learning in mice bred for increased voluntary wheel running." *Behavioral Neuroscience* 2003; 117(5): 1006–16.

Van Praag, H, et al. "Exercise enhances learning and hippocampal neurogenesis in aged mice." *Soc Neuroscience* 2008; 25(38): 8680–5.

Voss, M, et al. "Exercise, brain, and cognition across the life span." *J Appl Physiol* 2011; 111(5): 1505–13.

Walberg, J. "Aerobic exercise and resistance

weight-training during weight reduction, Implications for obese persons and athletes." *Sports Med* 1989; 7(6):343–56.

Wenk, G, et al. "Neurotransmitters and memory: Role of cholinergic, serotonergic, and noradrenergic systems." *Behav Neurosci* 1987; 101(3):325–32.

Chapter 9: Mental Activity

Ball, K. "Effects of cognitive training with older adults." *JAMA* 2002; 288(18): 2271–81.

Barnes, D, et al. "The mental activity and eXercise (MAX) trial: a randomized controlled trial to enhance cognitive function in older adults." *JAMA Intern Med* 2013; 173(9):797–804.

Bassuk, S, et al. "Social disengagement and incident cognitive decline in community-dwelling elderly persons." *Ann Int Med* 1999; 131(3): 165–73.

Breuil, V, et al. "Cognitive stimulation of patients with dementia; preliminary results." *J Ger Psychiatry* 1994; 9(3): 211–7.

Cacioppo, J, and L Hawkley. "Perceived social isolation and cognition." *Trends Cog Sci* 2009; 13(10): 447–54.

Chan, A, et al. "Music training improves verbal memory." *Nature* 1998; 396(6707):128.

Cotman, C. "Synaptic plasticity, neurotrophic factors, and transplantation in the aged brain." In *Handbook of the Biology of Aging*, edited by Edward Schneider, 225–74. San Diego, CA: Academic Press, 1990.

Diamond, M., et al. "Differences in occipital cortical synapses from environmentally enriched, impoverished, and standard colony rats." *J Neurosci Res* 1975; 1(2):109–19.

Ertel, K, et al. "Effects of social integration on preserving memory function in a nationally representative US elderly population." *Am J Pub Health* 2008; 98(7): 1215–20.

Fratiglioni, L. "An active and socially integrated lifestyle in late life might protect against dementia." *Lancet Neurol* 2004; 3:343–53.

Fratiglioni, L, et al. "Brain reserve hypothesis in dementia." *J Alzheimer's Dis* 2007; 12(1):11–22.

Glass, T, et al. "Population based study of social and productive activities as predictors of survival among elderly Americans." *BMJ* 1999; 319(7208): 478–83.

Goldman, R. *Brain Fitness.* New York: Doubleday, 1998.

"Healthy brain aging: no strain, no gain." *Harvard Men's Health Watch* 2012; 17(4):3.

Jak, A. "The impact of physical and mental activity on cognitive aging." *Curr Top Behav Neurosci* 2012; 10:273–91.

Pinquart, M, et al. "Influences of socioeconomic status, social network, and competence on subjective well-being in later life: a meta-analysis." *Psychol Aging* 2000; 15(2): 187–224.

Salthouse, T. "Mental exercise and mental aging: evaluating the validity of the 'Use it or Lose it' hypothesis." *Persp Psychol Sci* 2006; 1(1): 68–87.

Schweizer, T, et al. "Bilingualism as a contributor to cognitive reserve: evidence from brain atrophy in Alzheimer's disease." *Cortex* 2012; 48(8):991–6.

Seeman, T. "Social ties and health: the benefits of social integration." *Ann Epidemiol* 1996; 6(5):442–51.

Valenzuela, M, et al. "Brain reserve and dementia: a systematic review." *Psychol Med* 2006; 36(4):441–54.

Wang, H, et al. "Late-life engagement in social and leisure activities is associated with a decreased risk of dementia: a longitudinal study from the Kungsholmen project." *Am J Epidemiol* 2002: 155(12): 1081–7.

Willis, S, et al. "Long-term effects of cognitive training on everyday functional outcomes in older adults." *JAMA* 2006; 296(23):2805–14.

Zatorre, R. "Music, the food of neuroscience?" *Nature* 2005; 434(7031):312–5.

Chapter 10: Sleep

Centers for Disease Control. "Sleep hygiene tips." Last modified March 13, 2013. www.cdc.gov/sleep/about_sleep/sleep_hygiene.htm.

Division of Sleep Medicine at Harvard Medical School. "Twelve simple tips to improve your sleep." Last modified December 18, 2007. http://healthysleep.med.harvard.edu/healthy/getting/overcoming/tips.

Gaby, A. *Nutritional Medicine.* Concord, NH: Fritz Perlberg Publishing, 2011.

Okawa, M, et al. "Vitamin B12 treatment for delayed sleep phase syndrome: a multi-center double-blind study." *Psychiatry Clin Neurosci* 1997; 51(5):275–9.

—. "Vitamin B12 treatment for sleep-wake rhythm disorders." *Sleep* 1190; 13(1):15–23.

Roberts, H. "Reactions attributed to aspartame-containing products: 551 cases." *J Appl Nutr* 1988; 40(8):5–94.

Smith, P. *What You Must Know About Vitamins, Minerals, Herbs, and More.* Garden City Park, NY: Square One Publishers, 2008.

Speroni, E., et al. "Neuropharmacological activity of extracts from Passiflora incarnate," Planta Med 1988; 488–91.

University of Maryland Medical Center. "Sleep hygiene." Last modified July 31, 2013. http://umm.edu/programs/sleep/patients/sleep-hygiene.

Chapter 11: Stress Management

Centers for Disease Control. "Managing stress." Last modified December 19, 2012. www.cdc.gov/features/handlingstress.

Mayo Clinic. "Stress management." Last modified March 19, 2011. www.mayoclinic.com/health/stress-management/MY00435.

National Library of Medicine. "Stress management." Last modified October 23, 2012. www.nlm.nih.gov/medlineplus/ency/article/001942.htm.

Chapter 12: Diet

Carrera-Bastos, P, et al. "The western diet and lifestyle and diseases of civilization." *Res Rep Clin Cardiol* 2011; 2:15–35.

Féart, C, et al. "Adherence to a Mediterranean Diet, cognitive decline, and risk of dementia." *JAMA* 2009; 302(6):638–48.

Harvard School of Public Health. "Health gains from whole grains." Accessed October 4, 2013. www.hsph.harvard.edu/nutritionsource/what-should-you-eat/health-gains-from-whole-grains/.

Kankowa, K. "Diabetic threesome (hyperglycemia, renal function, and nutrition) and advanced glycation end products: evidence for the multiple-hit agent?" *Proc Nutr Soc* 2008; 67(1): 60–74.

Kaur, H, et al. "Protective effect of lycopene on oxidative stress and cognitive decline in rotenone induced model of Parkinson's disease." *Neurochem Res* 2011; 36(8):1435–43.

Scarmeas, N. "Mediterranean diet and risk for Alzheimer's disease." *Ann Neurol* 2006; 59(6): 912–21.

—. "Mediterranean diet and mild cognitive impairment." *Arch Neurol* 2009; 66(2): 216–25.

Sofi, F. "Adherence to Mediterranean diet and health status: meta-analysis." *BMJ* 2008; 337.

Solfrizzi, V, et al. "The role of diet in cognitive decline." *J Neural Transm* 2003; 110:95–110.

Trichopoulou, A. "Anatomy of health effects of Mediterranean diet: Greek EPIC prospective cohort study." *BMJ* 2009; 338:b2337.

Uribarri, J, et al. "Advanced glycation products in foods and a practical guide to the reduction in the diet." *J Am Diet Assoc* 2010; 110(6): 911–16e12.

Willett, W, et al. "Mediterranean diet pyramid: a cultural model for healthy eating." *Am J Clin Nutr* 1995; 61(6):14025–165.

Chapter 13: Supplements

Abalan, F, and J Delile. "B12 deficiency in presenile dementia." *Biol Psychiatry* 1985; 20(11):1251.

Aisen, P, et al. "High-dose B vitamin supplementation and cognitive decline in Alzheimer's disease: a randomized controlled trial." *JAMA* 2008; 300(15):1774–83.

Akhondzadeh, S, et al. "Melissa officinalis etract in the treatment of patients with mild to moderate Alzheimer's disease: a double-blind, randomized, placebo-controlled trial." *J Neurol Neurosurg Psychiatry* 2003; 74(7):863–6.

Allegro, L, et al. "Oral phosphatidylserine in elderly patients with cognitive deterioration: an open study." *Clin Trials J* 1987; 24(1):104–8.

Amaducci, L. "Phosphatidylserine in the treatment of Alzheimer's disease: results of multicenter study." *Psychopharmacol Bull* 1988; 24(1):130–4.

Arterburn, L, et al. "Algal-oil capsules and cooked salmon: nutritionally equivalent sources of docosahexaenoic acid." *J Am Diet Assoc* 2008; 108(7):1204–9.

—. "Bioequivalence of docosahexaenoic acid from different algal oils in capsules and in a DHA-fortified food." *Lipids* 2007; 41(11): 1011–24.

—. "Distribution, interconversion, and dose response of n-3 fatty acids in humans." *Am J Clin Nutr* 2006; 83(6 Suppl):1467S-76S.

Balu, M, et al. "Modulatory role of grape seed extract on age-related oxidative DHA damage in central nervous system of rats." *Brain Res Bull* 2006; 68(6):469–73.

Barak, Y, et al. "Inositol treatment of Alzheimer's disease: a double-blind, cross-over placebo controlled trial." *Prog Neuropsychopharmacol Biol Psychiatry* 1996; 20(4):729–35.

Bazan, N. "Neuroprotectin D1 (NPD1): a DHA-derived mediator that protects brain and retina against cell injury-induced oxidative stress." *Brain Pathol* 2005; 15(2):159–66.

—. "The onset of brain injury and neurodegeneration triggers the synthesis of docosanoid neuroprotective signaling." *Cell Mol Neurobiol* 2006; 26(4–6):901–13.

Bazan, N, et al. "Brain response to injury and neurodegeneration: endogenous neuroprotective signaling." *Ann NY Acad Sci* 2005; 1053: 137–47.

—. "Docosahexaenoic acid signalolipidomics in nutrition, significance in aging, neuroinflammation, macular degeneration, Alzheimer's and other neurodegenerative diseases." *Ann Rev Nutr* 2011; 31:321–51.

—. "Endogenous signaling by omega-3-docosahexaenoic acid-derived mediators sustains homeostatic synaptic and circuitry integrity." *Mol Neurobiol* 2011; 44(2):216–22.

Behl, C, et al. "Vitamin E protects nerve cells from amyloid beta protein toxicity." *Biochem Biophys Res Commun* 1992; 186(2):944–50.

Birkmayer, J. "Coenzyme nicotinamide adenine dinucleotide. New therapeutic approach for improving dementia of the Alzheimer type." *Ann Clin Lab Sci* 1996; 26(1):1–9.

Birks, J, and J Grimley Evans. "Ginkgo biloba for cognitive impairment and dementia." *Cochrane Databse Syst Rev* 2007; 18(2):CD003120.

Bonavita, E. "Study of the efficacy and tolerability of L-acetyl carnitine therapy in the senile brain." *Int Jour Clin Pharmacol Ther Toxicol* 1986; 24(9):511–6.

Bönöczk, P, et al. "Role of sodium channel inhibition in neuroprotection: effect of vinpocetine." *Brain Res Bull* 2000; 53(3):245–54.

Bowman, B. "Acetyl-L-carnitine and Alzheimer's disease." *Nutr Rev* 1992; 50(5):142–4.

Bradbury, J. "Docosahexaenoic acid (DHA): an ancient nutrient for the modern human brain." *Nutrients* 2011; 3(5):529–54.

Brooks, J, et al. "Acetyl-L-carnitine slows decline in younger patients with Alzheimer's disease: a reanalysis of a double-blind, placebo-controlled study using the trilinear approach." *Int Psychogeriatr* 1998; 10(2):192–203.

Buchman, A, et al. "Verbal and visual memory improvement after choline supplementation in long-term total parenteral nutrition: a pilot study." *J Parenter Enteral Nutr* 2001; 25(1):30–5.

Burnet, F. "A possible role of zinc in the pathology of dementia." Lancet 1981; 1(8213):186–8.

Burns, A, and T Holland. "Vitamin E deficiency." *Lancet* 1992; 327(8484):805–6.

Caffarra, P, and V Santamaria. "The effects of phosphatidylserine in patients with mild cognitive decline: an open trial." *Clin Trial J* 1987; 24(1):109–14.

Calvani, M, et al. "Action of acetyl-L-carnitine in neurodegeneration and Alzheimer's disease." *Ann NY Acad Sci* 1992; 663:483–6.

Cao, D, et al. "Docosahexaenoic acid promotes hippocampal neuronal development and synaptic function." *J Neurochem* 2009; 111(2): 510–21.

Carta, A, et al. "Acetyl-L-carnitine and Alzheimer's disease: pharmacological considerations beyond the cholinergic sphere." *Ann NY Acad Sci* 1993; 695:324–6.

Castorina, M, et al. "Acetyl-L-carnitine affects

aged brain receptorial system in rodents." *Life Sci* 1994; 54(17):1205–14.

Cenacchi, T, et al. "Cognitive decline in the elderly: a double-blind, placebo-controlled multicenter study on efficacy of phosphatidylserine administration." *Aging: Clin Exper Res* 1993; 5(2):123–33.

Cole, G, and S Frautschy. "Docosahexaenoic acid protects from amyloid and dendritic pathology in an Alzheimer's disease mouse model." *Nutr Health* 2006; 18(3):249–59.

Cole, M, et al. "Low serum vitamin B12 in Alzheimer-type dementia." *Age Ageing* 1984; 13(2):101–5.

Constantinidis, J. "The hypothesis of zinc deficiency in the pathogenesis of neurofibrillary tangles." *Med Hypoth* 1991; 35(4):319–23.

Constantinidis, J, et al. "Treatment of Alzheimer's disease by zinc compounds." *Drug Dev Res* 1992; 27(1):1–14.

Cucinotta, D, et al. "Multicenter clinical placebo-controlled study with acetyl-L-carnitine (LAC) in the treatment of mildly demented elderly patients." *Drug Dev Res* 1988; 14(3–4): 213–6.

Defeudis, F. *Ginkgo biloba extract (Egb 761): Pharmacological Activities and Clinical Applications.* Paris: Elsevier, 1991.

Deijen, J, et al. "Vitamin B6 supplementation in elderly men: effects on mood, memory, performance and mental effort." *Psychopharmacology* 1992; 109(4):489–96.

De Jesus Moreno, M. "Cognitive improvement in mild to moderate Alzheimer's dementia after treatment with acetylcholine precursor alfoscerate: a multicenter, double-blind, placebo-controlled trial." *Clin Ther* 2003; 25(1):178–93.

Delwaide, P, et al. "Double-blind randomized controlled study of phosphatidylserine in senile demented patients." *Acta Neurol Scand* 1986; 73(2):136–40.

Demarin, V, et al. "Treatment of Alzheimer's disease with stabilized oral nicotinamide adenine dinucleotide: a randomized, double-blind study." *Drugs Exp Clin Res* 2004; 30(1):27–33.

Dos Santos-Neto, et al. "The use of herbal medicine in Alzheimer's disease—a systemic review." *Evid Based Complement Alternat Med* 2006; 3(4):441–5.

Drachman, D. "Memory and cognitive function in man: does the cholinergic system have a specific role?" *Neurology* 1977; 27(8):783–90.

Durga, F, et al. "Effect of 3-year folic acid supplementation on cognitive function in older adults in the FACIT trial: a randomized, double-blind, controlled trial." *Lancet* 2007; 369(9557):208–16.

Engelhart, M, et al. "Dietary intake of antioxidants and risk of Alzheimer disease." *JAMA* 2002; 287(24):3223–9.

Enk, C, et al. "Reversible dementia and neuropathy associated with folate deficiency 16 years after partial gastrectomy." *Scand J Haematol* 1980; 25(6):63–6.

Ernst, E, and M Pittler. "Ginkgo biloba for dementia: a systematic review of double-blind, placebo-controlled trials." *Clin Drug Investig* 1999; 17:301–8.

Etienne, P, et al. "Clinical effects of choline in Alzheimer's disease," *Lancet* 1978; 311(8062): 508–9.

Eussen, S, et al. "Effect of oral vitamin B12 with or without folic acid on cognitive function in older people with mild vitamin B12 deficiency: a randomized, placebo-controlled trial." *Am J Clin Nutr* 2006; 84(2):361–70.

Fekkes, D, et al. "Abnormal amino acid metabolism in patients with early stage Alzheimer's dementia." *J Neural Transm* 1998; 105(2–3): 287–94.

Ferris, S, et al. "Long-term choline treatment of memory-impaired elderly patients." *Science* 1979; 205(4410):1039–40.

Forsyth, L, et al. "Therapeutic effects of oral NADH on symptoms of patients with chronic fatigue syndrome." *Ann Allergy Asthma Immunol* 1999; 82(2):185–91.

Freyre, A, and J Flichman. "Spasmophilia caused by magnesium deficit." *Psychosomatics* 1970; 11(5):500–1.

Gaby, A. *Nutritional Medicine.* Concord, NH: Fritz Perlberg Publishing, 2011.

Gibson, G, et al. "Reduced activities of thiamine-dependent enzymes in the brains and peripheral tissues of patients with Alzheimer's disease." *Arch Neurol* 1988; 45(8):836–40.

Gold, M, et al. "Plasma and red blood cell thiamine deficiency in patients with dementia of the Alzheimer's type." *Arch Neurol* 1995; 52(11):1081–6.

Granata, Q, and J DiMichele. "Phosphatidylserine in elderly patients: an open trial." *Clin Trials J* 1987; 24(1):99–103.

Grodstein, F, et al. "A randomized trial of beta carotene supplementation and cognitive function in men: the Physicians' Health Study II." *Arch Inter Med* 2007; 167(20):2184–90.

He, C, et al. "Improved spatial learning performance of fat-1 mice is associated with enhanced neurogenesis and neuritogenesis by docosahexaenoic acid." *Pro Natl Acad Sci USA* 2009; 106(27):11370–5.

Hector, M, and J Burton. "What are the psychiatric manifestations of vitamin B12 deficiency?" *J Am Geriatr Soc* 1988; 36(12):1105–12.

Heiss, W, et al. "Long-term effects of phosphatidylserine, pyritinol, and cognitive training in Alzheimer's disease," *Dementia* 1994; 5(2):88–98.

Hoffer, A. "Senility and chronic malnutrition." *J Orthomol Psychiatry* 1974; 3:2–19.

Horning, M, et al. "Endogenous mechanisms of neuroprotection: role of zinc, copper, and carnosine." *Brain Res* 2000; 852(1):56–61.

Horrocks, L, and Y Yeo. "Health benefits of docosahexaenoic acid (DHA)." *Pharmacol Res* 1999; 40(3):211–25.

Huguet, F, et al. "Decreased cerebral 5-HTIA receptors during aging: reversal by Ginkgo biloba extract (EGb 761)." *J Pharm Pharmacol* 1994; 46(4):316–8.

Jorissen, B, et al. "The influence of soy-derived phosphatidylserine on cognition in age-associated memory impairment." *Nutr Neurosci* 2001; 4(2):121–34.

Kanofsky, J. "Thiamine status and cognitive impairment in the elderly." *J Am Coll Nutr* 1996; 15(3):197–8.

Kanowski, S, et al. "Proof of efficacy of the Ginkgo biloba special extract EGb 761 in outpatients suffering from mild to moderate primary degenerative dementia of the Alzheimer type or multi-infarct dementia of the Alzheimer type or multi-infarct dementia." *Pharmacopsychiatry* 1996; 29(2):47–56.

Kidd, P. *Phosphatidylserine: Nature's Brain Booster for Memory, Mood, and Stress.* St. George, UT: Total Health Communications, Inc., 2007.

Klatte, E, et al. "Combination therapy of donepezil and vitamin E in Alzheimer disease." *Alzheimer Dis Assoc Disord* 2003; 17(2):113–6.

Kleijnen, J, and P Knipschild. "Ginkgo biloba." *Lancet* 1992; 340(8828):1136–9.

Kristensen, M, et al. "Serum cobalamin and methylmalonic acid in Alzheimer dementia." *Acta Neurol Scand* 1993; 87(6):475–81.

Kuboyama, T, et al. "Neuritic regeneration and synaptic reconstruction induced by withanolide A." *Brit J Pharmacol* 2005; 144(7):961–71.

Kyle, D, et al. "Low serum docosahexaenoic acid is a significant risk factor for Alzheimer's dementia." *Lipids* 1999; 34 (Suppl):S245.

Lakhani, S, et al. "Small intestinal bacterial overgrowth and thiamine deficiency after Roux-en-Y gastric bypass surgery in obese patients." *Nutr Res* 2008; 28(5):293–8.

Lange, K, and M Mahl. "A long-term study of the effect of nicotinic acid medication on hypercholesterolemia." *Am J Med Sci* 1963; 246: 673–77.

Le Bars, P, et al. "A placebo-controlled, double-blind, randomized trial of an extract of Ginkgo biloba for dementia." *JAMA* 1997; 278(16): 1327–32.

Lehmann, J, et al. "Tryptophan malabsorption in dementia. Improvement in certain cases after tryptophan therapy as indicated by mental behavior and blood analysis." *Acta Psychiatr Scand* 1981; 64(2):123–31.

Lemke, M. "Plasma magnesium decrease and altered calcium/magnesium ratio in severe dementia of the Alzheimer type." *Biol Psychiatry* 1995; 37(5):341–3.

Levy, R, et al. "Early results from double-blind, placebo-controlled trial of high-dose phosphatidylcholine in Alzheimer's disease." *Lancet* 1983; 321(8331):987–8.

Li, M, et al. "Protective effects of oligomers of grape seed polyphenols against beta-amyloid-induced oxidative cell death." *Ann NY Acad Sci* 2004; 1030:317–29.

Martin, D, et al. "Time dependency of cognitive recovery with cobalamin replacement. A report of a pilot study." *J Am Geriatr Soc* 1992; 40(2): 168–72.

Masaki, K, et al. "Association of vitamin E and C supplement use with cognitive function and dementia in elderly men." *Neurology* 2000; 54(6):1265–72.

McCann, J, et al. "Is docosahexaenoic acid, an n-3 long-chain polyunsaturated fatty acid, required for development of normal brain function? An overview of evidence from cognitive and behavioral tests in humans and animals." *Am J Clin Nutr* 2005; 82(2):281–95.

McDaniel, M, et al. "Brain-specific nutrients: a memory cure?" *Nutrition* 2003; 19(11–12): 957–75.

Meador, K, et al. "Evidence for a central cholinergic effect of high-dose thiamine." *Ann Neurol* 1993; 34(5):724–6.

—. "Preliminary findings of high-dose thiamine in dementia of Alzheimer's type," *J Geriatr Psychiatry Neurol* 1993; 6(4):222–9.

Mimori, Y, et al. "Thiamine therapy in Alzheimer's disease." *Metab Brain Dis* 1996; 11(1):89–94.

Mitsuyama, Y, et al. "Serum and cerebrospinal fluid vitamin B12 levels in demented patients with CH3-B12 treatment—preliminary study." *Jpn J Psychiatry Neurol* 1988; 42(1):65–71.

Monteleone, P, et al. "Effects of phosphatidyl-serine on the neuroendocrine response to physical stress in humans." *Neuroendocrinology* 1990; 52(3):243–8.

Mohs, R, et al. "Choline chloride treatment of memory deficits in the elderly." *Am J Psychiatry* 1979; 136(10):1275–7.

Morris, MC, et al. "Consumption of fish and n-3 fatty acids and risk of incident Alzheimer disease." *Arch Neurol* 2003; 60(7):940–6.

—. "Dietary intake of antioxidant nutrients and the risk of incident Alzheimer disease in a biracial community study." *JAMA* 2002; 287(24): 3230–7.

—. Morris, M, et al. "Relation of the tocopherol forms to incident Alzheimer disease and to cognitive change." *Am J Clin Nutr* 2005; 81(2): 508–14.

—. "Vitamin E and vitamin C supplement use and risk of incident Alzheimer disease." *Alzheimer Dis Assoc Disord* 1998; 12(3):121–6.

Morris, M, et al. "Hyperhomocysteinemia associated with poor recall in the third National Health and Nutrition Examination Survey." *Am J Clin Nutr* 2001; 73(5):927–33.

Nolan, K, et al. "A trial of thiamine in Alzheimer's disease." *Arch Neurol* 1991; 48(1): 81–3.

Packer, L. "Alpha-lipoic acid: a metabolic antioxidant which regulates NF-kappa B signal transduction and protects against oxidative injury." *Drug Metabol Rev* 1998; 30(2):245–75.

Packer, L, et al. "Neuroprotection by the metabolic antioxidant alpha-lipoic acid." *Free Radic Biol Med* 1997; 22(1–2):359–78.

Papandreou, M, et al. "Effect of polyphenol-rich wild blueberry extract on cognitive performance of mice, brain antioxidant markers, and acetylcholinesterase activity." *Behav Brain Res* 2008; 198(2):352–8.

Passeri, M, et al. "Acetyl-L-carnitine in the treatment of mildly demented elderly patients." *Int Jour of Clin Pharmacol Res* 1988; 8(5):367–78.

Pettegrew, J, et al. "Clinical and neurochemical effects of acetyl-L-carnitine in Alzheimer's disease." *Neurobiol Aging* 1995; 16(1):1–4.

Potocnik, F, et al. "Zinc and platelet membrane microviscosity in Alzheimer's disease. The in vivo effect of zinc on platelet membranes and cognition." *S Afr Med J* 1997; 87(9):1116–9.

Puca, F, et al. "Exploratory trial of phosphatidylserine efficacy in mildly demented patients." *Clin Trials J* 1987; 24:94–8.

Rai, G, et al. "Double-blind placebo controlled study of acetyl-L-carnitine in patients with Alzheimer's dementia." *Curr Med Res Opin* 1990; 11(10):638–47.

Ravaglia, G, et al. "Homocysteine and folate as risk factors for dementia and Alzheimer's disease." *Am J Clin Nutr* 2005; 82(3):636–43.

Regland, B, et al. "Low B12 levels related to high activity of platelet MAO in patients with dementia disorders. A retrospective study." *Acta Pychiatr Scand* 1988; 78(4):451–7.

—. "Vitamin B12 in CSF: reduced CSF/serum B12 ratio in demented men." *Acta Neurol Scand* 1992; 85(4):276–81.

Renvoize, E, and T Jerram. "Choline in Alzheimer's disease." *NEJM* 1979; 301(6):330.

Riedel, W, et al. "Tryptophan depletion in normal volunteers produces selective impairment in memory consolidation." *Psychopharmacology* 1999; 141(4):362–9.

Rondanelli, M, et al. "Effects of a diet integration with an oily emulsion of DHA-phospholipids containing melatonin and tryptophan in elderly patients suffering from mild cognitive impairment." *Nutr Neurosci* 2012; 15(2):46–54.

Salvioli, G, and M Neri. "L-acetyl carnitine treatment of mental decline in the elderly," *Drugs Exp Clin Res* 1994; 20(4):169–76.

Sanchez, C, et al. "The relationship between dietary intake of choline, choline serum levels, and cognitive function in healthy elderly persons." *J Am Geriatr Soc* 1984; 32(3):209–12.

Sanders, T, et al. "DHA status of vegetarians," *Prostaglandins Leukot Essent Fatty Acids* 2009; 81(2–3):137–41.

Sano, M, et al. "A controlled trial of selegiline, alpha-tocopherol, or both as treatment for Alzheimer's disease: the Alzheimer's Disease Cooperative Study." *NEJM* 1997; 336(17): 1216–22.

—. "Double-blind parallel design pilot study of acetyl levocarnitine in patients with Alzheimer's disease." *Arch Neurol* 1992; 49(11):1137–41.

Sapira, J, et al. "Reversible dementia due to folate deficiency." *S Med J* 1975; 68(6):776–7.

Sen, C, et al. "Molecular basis of vitamin E action: tocotrienol potently inhibits glutamate-induced pp60c-Src kinase activation and death of HT4 neuronal cells." *J Biol Chemistry* 2000; 275(17):13049–55.

Seshadri, S, et al. "Plasma homocysteine as a risk factor for dementia and Alzheimer's disease." *NEJM* 2002; 346(7):476–83.

Shaw, D, et al. "Pilot study of amino acids in senile dementia." *Br J Psychiatry* 1981; 139:580–2.

Shevell, M, et al. "The neurology of cobalamin." *Cam J Neurol Sci* 1992; 19(4):472–86.

Sinforiani, E, et al. "Cognitive decline in ageing brain. Therapeutic approach with phosphatidylserine." *Clin Trials J* 1987; 24(1):115–24.

Sinn, N, et al. "Effects of n-3 fatty acids. EPA vs DHA, on depressive symptoms, quality of life, memory and executive function in older adults with mild cognitive impairment: a 6-month randomized controlled trial." *Brit J Nutr* 2012; 107(11):1682–93.

SMID Group. "Phosphatidylserine in the treatment of clinically diagnosed Alzheimer's disease." *J Neural Transm* 1987; 24(Suppl):287–92.

Smith, D, et al. "Lack of effect of tryptophan treatment in demented gerontopsychiatric patients." *Acta Psychiatr Scan* 1984; 70(5): 470–7.

Spagnoli, A, et al. "Long-term acetyl-L-carnitine treatment of Alzheimer's disease." *Neurology* 1991; 41(11):1726–32.

Steiner, I, and E Melamed. "Folic acid and the nervous system." *Neurology* 1983; 33(12):1634.

Stokel, K. "DHA: an essential brain food." *Life Extension* Nov. 2012, 66–73.

Szilágyi, G, et al. "Effects of vinpocetine on the redistribution of cerebral blood flow and glucose metabolism in chronic ischemic stroke patients: a PET study." *J Neurol Sci* 2005; 229–230:275–84.

Terano, T, et al. "Docosahexaenoic acid supplementation improves the moderately severe dementia from thrombotic cerebrovascular diseases." *Lipids* 1999; 34(1 Suppl):S345–6.

Thal, L, et al. "A 1-year controlled trial of acetyl-L-carnitine in early-onset Alzheimer's disease." *Neurology* 2000; 55(6):805–10.

Tucker, K, et al. "High homocysteine and low B vitamins predict cognitive decline in aging men: the Veterans Affairs Normative Aging Study." *Am J Clin Nutr* 2005; 82(3):627–35.

Tully, C, et al. "Serum zinc senile plaques and neurofibrillary tangles: findings from the Bun Study." *Neuroreport* 1995; 6(16):2105–8.

Van Goor, L, et al. "Review: cobalamin deficiency and mental impairment in elderly people." *Age Ageing* 1995; 24(6):536–42.

Van Tiggelen, C, et al. "Assessment of vitamin B12 status in CSF." *Am J Psychiatry* 1984; 141(1): 136–7.

Vecchi, G, et al., "Acetyl-L-carnitine treatment

of mental impairment in the elderly: evidence from a multicenter study." *Arch Gerontol Geriatr* 1991; 2(Supp 2):159–68.

Villardita, C, et al. "Multicentre clinical trial of brain phosphatidylserine in elderly patients with intellectual deterioration." *Clin Trials J* 1987; 24(1):84–93.

Wang, A, et al. "Use of carnosine as a natural anti-senescence drug for human beings," *Biochemistry* 2000; 65(7):869–71.

Watanabe, C, et al. "The in vivo neuromodulatory effects of the herbal medicine ginkgo biloba." *Proc Natl Acad Sci USA* 2001; 98(12): 6577–80.

Wettstein, A. "Cholinesterase inhibitors and ginkgo extracts—are they comparable in the treatment of dementia? Comparison of published placebo-controlled efficacy studies of at least six months' duration." *Phytomedicine* 2000; 6(6):383–401.

Xu, S, et al. "Efficacy of tablet huperzine-A on memory, cognition, and behavior in Alzheimer's disease." *Zhongguo Yao Li Xue Bao* 1995; 16(5):391–95.

Yao, A, et al. "Ginkgo biloba extract (EGb 761) inhibits beta-amyloid production by lowering free cholesterol levels." *J Nutr Biochem* 2004; 15(12):749–56.

Ying, W. "NAD+ and NADH in brain functions, brain diseases and brain aging." *Front Biosci* 2007; 12:1863–88.

—. "NAD+/NADH and NADP+/NADPH in cellular functions and cell death: regulation and biological consequences." *Antioxid Redox Signal* 2008; 10(2):179–206.

Zaman, Z, et al. "Plasma concentrations of vitamins A and E and carotenoids in Alzheimer's disease." *Age Ageing* 1992; 21(2):91–4.

Zandi, P, et al. "Reduced risk of Alzheimer disease in users of antioxidant vitamin supplements: the Cache County Study." *Arch Neurol* 2004; 61(1):82–8.

Zhang, H, et al. "Non-cholinergic effects of huperzine A: beyond inhibition of acetylcholinesterase." *Cell Mol Neurobiol* 2008; 28(2): 173–83.

About the Author

Pamela Wartian Smith, MD, MPH, MS, is a diplomate of the American Academy of Anti-Aging Physicians and director of the Master's Program in Medical Sciences, with a concentration in Metabolic and Nutritional Medicine, at the University of South Florida College of Medicine. An authority on the subjects of wellness and anti-aging, Dr. Smith is also co-director of the Fellowship in Anti-Aging, Regenerative, and Functional Medicine. Currently, she is the owner and co-director of the Center for Healthy Living, with locations in Michigan and Florida. Dr. Smith is the best-selling author of *What You Must Know About Vitamins, Minerals, Herbs & More; What You Must Know About Women's Hormones;* and *Why You Can't Lose Weight.*

Index

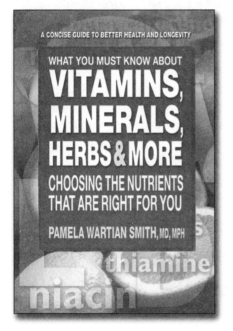

WHAT YOU MUST KNOW ABOUT VITAMINS, MINERALS, HERBS & MORE

Choosing the Nutrients
That Are Right for You

Pamela Wartian Smith, MD, MPH

Almost 75 percent of your health and life expectancy is based on lifestyle, environment, and nutrition. Yet even if you follow a healthful diet, you are probably not getting all the nutrients you need to prevent disease. In *What You Must Know About Vitamins, Minerals, Herbs & More,* Dr. Pamela Smith explains how to determine which nutrients are right for you, and how nutrient deficiencies can lead to chronic disease.

Part 1 of this easy-to-use guide provides the individual nutrients necessary for good health. In Part 2, it offers personalized nutritional programs for people with a wide variety of illnesses and disorders. People without prior medical problems—men, women, vegetarians, smokers, dieters, and more—can look to Part 3 for their supplementation plans. Whether you want to maintain good health or are trying to overcome a medical condition, *What You Must Know About Vitamins, Minerals, Herbs & More* can help you make the best choices for your diet and supplementation program.

$15.95 US • 448 pages • 6 x 9-inch quality paperback • ISBN 978-0-7570-0233-5

WHAT YOU MUST KNOW ABOUT WOMEN'S HORMONES

Your Guide to Natural Hormone Treatments for PMS, Menopause, Osteoporosis, PCOS, and More

Pamela Wartian Smith, MD, MPH

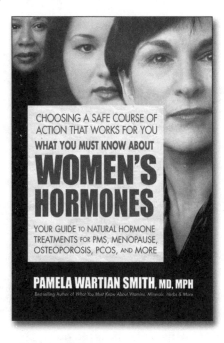

Hormonal imbalances can occur at any age—before, during, or after menopause. The reason for these imbalances vary widely, and can include heredity, environment, nutrition, and aging. While most hormone-related problems are associated with menopause, the fact is that fluctuating hormonal levels can also cause a variety of other conditions, and for some women, the effects can be truly debilitating. *What You Must Know About Women's Hormones* is a clear and concise guide to the treatment of hormonal irregularities without the health risks associated with standard hormone replacement therapy.

This book is divided into three parts. Part I describes the body's own hormones, looking at their functions and the different side effects that can occur if these hormones are not at optimal levels. Part II focuses on the most common problems that arise from hormonal imbalances, such as PMS, hot flashes, postpartum depression, and endometriosis. You will learn that even disorders that seemingly have nothing to do with hormones, such as heart disease and osteoporosis, can be affected by a hormonal imbalance. Lastly, Part III details hormone replacement therapy, focusing on the difference between natural and synthetic hormone treatments. It explains how you can have your hormonal levels measured, and provides examples of the various hormone replacement therapies available.

Whether you are looking for help with menopausal symptoms or you simply want to enjoy vibrant health, *What You Must Know About Women's Hormones* can make a profound difference in the quality of your life.

$17.95 US • 256 pages • 6 x 9-inch quality paperback • ISBN 978-0-7570-0307-3

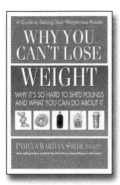

WHY YOU CAN'T LOSE WEIGHT
Why It's So Hard to Shed Pounds and What You Can Do About It

Pamela Wartian Smith, MD, MPH

If you have tried diet after diet without shedding pounds, it may not be your fault. In this revolutionary book, Dr. Pamela Smith discusses the eighteen most common reasons why you can't lose weight, and guides you in overcoming the obstacles that stand between you and a trimmer body.

Why You Can't Lose Weight is divided into four parts. Part I looks at lifestyle practices, such as insufficient exercise and sleep. Part II examines health disorders, such as food allergies and thyroid hormone dysfunction. And Part III discusses biochemical problems, such as insulin resistance and depression. For each difficulty discussed, the author explains how the problem can be recognized, how it contributes to weight gain, and how you can take steps towards a slimmer body. The last part guides you in putting together a customized, easy-to-follow weight-loss program.

If you've been frustrated by one-size-fits-all diet plans, it's time to learn what's really keeping you from reaching your goal. With *Why You Can't Lose Weight,* you'll discover how to lose weight and enjoy radiant health.

$16.95 US • 256 pages • 6 x 9-inch quality paperback • ISBN 978-0-7570-0312-7

BITE IT & WRITE IT!
A Guide to Keeping Track of What You Eat & Drink

Stacie Castle, RD, Robyn Cotler, RD,
Marni Schefter, RD, and Shana Shapiro, RD

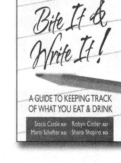

Professionals know that keeping track of what you eat and drink is the most effective way to improve your dietary habits. Designed by four nutritionists who have successfully used this system in their practices, *Bite It & Write It!* combines a structured food journal with an easy-to-follow nutrition guide.

Bite It & Write It! presents ten health goals—one for each week of the journal—and lets you record your daily food consumption as you work toward your objective. To help you along the way, the authors supply a wealth of nutritional information that will empower you to change the way you think about food and make a new commitment to improving your health. With this guide, you can track your calories, carbs, sodium, and water; record exercise; learn how to plan and prepare meals; and navigate restaurant menus without blowing your diet.

Whether your goal is to lose weight, manage a health problem, or simply feel better than you have in years, *Bite It & Write It!* can be your key to success.

$7.95 US • 192 pages • 4 x 7-inch mass paperback • ISBN 978-0-7570-0343-1

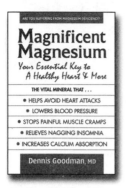

MAGNIFICENT MAGNESIUM
Your Essential Key to a Healthy Heart & More

Dennis Goodman, MD

Despite the development of many "breakthrough" drugs designed to combat its effects, heart disease remains the number-one killer of Americans. Is there a simpler solution? The answer is *yes*. For many years, scientists and medical researchers have known about a common mineral that can effectively prevent or remedy many cardiovascular conditions. And unlike the pharmaceuticals usually prescribed, this supplement has no dangerous side effects. In this book, world-renowned cardiologist Dr. Dennis Goodman shines a spotlight on magnesium, the mineral that can maximize your heart health.

Many drugs are designed to relieve the symptoms of heart disease, but none of them eliminates the root cause of the problem. In *Magnificent Magnesium*, you will discover how a simple all-natural mineral can improve the function of your heart and help you regain control of your health.

$14.95 US • 192 pages • 6 x 9-inch quality paperback • ISBN 978-0-7570-0391-2

YOUR BLOOD NEVER LIES
How to Read a Blood Test for a Longer, Healthier Life

James B. LaValle, RPh, CCN

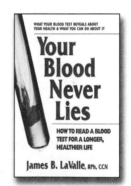

A standard blood test indicates how well the kidneys and liver are functioning, the potential for heart disease, and a host of other vital health markers. Unfortunately, most of us cannot decipher these results ourselves or even formulate the right questions to ask about them—or we couldn't, until now.

In *Your Blood Never Lies,* best-selling author James LaValle clears the mystery surrounding blood test results. In simple language, he explains all of the information found on these forms, making it understandable and accessible. This means that you can look at the results yourself and know the significance of each marker. Dr. LaValle even recommends the most effective treatments—both conventional and complementary—for dealing with any problematic findings. Rounding out the book are the names of test markers that should be requested for a more complete physical picture.

A blood test can reveal so much about your body, but only if you can interpret the results. *Your Blood Never Lies* provides the up-to-date information you need to take control of your health.

$16.95 US • 368 pages • 6 x 9-inch quality paperback • ISBN 978-0-7570-0350-9

For more information about our books,
visit our website at www.squareonepublishers.com